Integrated Teams in Primary Care

Edited by

Glyn Elwyn

and

June Smail

Forewords by

Denis Pereira Gray

and

Marion Bull

RADCLIFFE MEDICAL PRESS

Radcliffe Medical Press Ltd
18 Marcham Road, Abingdon, Oxon OX14 1AA, UK

British Library Cataloguing in Publication Data

A catalogue record for this book is available from the British Library.

ISBN 1 85775 288 0

Contents

Forewords   v

Preface   vii

List of contributors   ix

Acknowledgements   x

Introduction   1

Chapter 1   The changing organisation of primary care   7
Geoff Meads

Chapter 2   Integrated nursing teams and healthcare 'substitution'   13
Marcus Longley

Chapter 3   The political and policy context   27
Pippa Gough and Jonathan Richards

Chapter 4   Integrated nursing teams and the PHCT:
integral or alternative?   37
Glyn Elwyn and John Øvretveit

Chapter 5   Professional training issues for integrated
nursing teams   55
June Smail

Chapter 6   Nursing roles in integrated teams   67
Kate Harris

Chapter 7   Integrated nursing teams: sprouting up everywhere?   79
Peter Hodder

Chapter 8   Budgets and management: the Oxfordshire approach   91
Lisa Whordley and Jane Dauncey

Chapter 9   The legal aspects   101
             Bridgit Dimond

Chapter 10   Future directions for primary care   113
             Brenda Poulton

Index   125

Foreword

As primary care develops in a worldwide trend, so progressive interest is arising in who does what in primary care, with what effect, and at what cost.

Nurses are the most numerous of the health professionals now working in primary care and they have played a major part of its development in the UK. Primary care nursing has, however, been handicapped particularly by its training and its fragmentation, as there are as many as four quite different categories of nurses working in many primary care teams.

Issues of definition and objectives handicap the very term 'primary care team'. A classic study by Poulton and West (1993) showed that primary care teams often did not function well as judged by criteria of teamwork, and moreover were less developed than teams in other settings. That report and others stand as a challenge to all in primary care.

One obvious response is to seek to achieve better integration of the nursing presence within these teams, and there has been much thought about this and much written on the subject. This book brings the subject together; it is well referenced; and it tackles many of the outstanding issues. It is strong in charting the trends and showing how various health service reports and developments have influenced thinking. It is unusual in tackling new issues such as legal responsibility and devolved budgets, and includes practical examples.

Integrated Teams in Primary Care can be recommended to all those who wish to follow this important trend in primary care.

Denis Pereira Gray
General Practitioner, Exeter
Professor of General Practice, University of Exeter
President, Royal College of General Practitioners
September 1998

Foreword

This book is timely given the wide interest being shown in primary care organisations. Developments in primary care have stimulated all professionals to review their traditional ways of working. This has been done in my own profession under several banners – 'integrated nursing teams' and 'self-managed teams' being the terms used most frequently. The result has been that nurses, midwives and health visitors have recognised that primary care nursing requires colleagues with different skills to work together for a common purpose. To achieve such integration the nursing team requires strategies to overcome the barriers of poor communication and collaboration that have built up between nurses with different skills and different employers. These strategies will need to address the educational and professional development needs of primary care nursing and open up career pathways which recognise the value of the generalist approach in that primary care service. Such changes will need an organisational structure that facilitates this pooling of knowledge and skills to provide a flexible, effective and responsive nursing service within a multiprofessional primary care team.

The authors present an understanding of the context within which this change is taking place, the elements to be addressed in the change process and a challenge for the future direction and pace of change. A challenge which begins with a review of the traditional ways of working between nurses, and then extends to future working practices with other members of the primary care team. The reader is skilfully assisted to explore the prospect of this renewed emphasis on primary care organisations and their development with the benefit of authors and editors from a broad spectrum of opinion formers. The result is a thoughtful contribution to the literature and the debate on the way forward for some important aspects of primary care development.

Marion Bull
Chief Nursing Officer
Welsh Office
September 1998

Preface

The idea for this book emerged from two recent conferences in Wales and a number of seminars, workshops and lectures on integrated or practice-based nursing teams in the UK over the last year or two. A great deal of interest has been generated, particularly among nurses, about whether the concept of 'integration', and specifically 'integrated nursing teams', in primary care is just a passing phase or something which should be grasped and implemented.

To 'integrate' and 'the integration of' are commonly used words in today's NHS, meaning 'to bring into equal participation'. The fact that so many people are now interested in developing 'integrated teams in primary care' implies that there has been much dissatisfaction about the lack of integration between health visitors, district nurses, practice nurses and other primary care professionals in the past.

Although there is clear enthusiasm for developing integrated teams, it is also true to say that confusion and misunderstanding still exists. A number of articles on the subject have been published and various models implemented, mostly using a top-down approach, but no in-depth texts have been available to shed light on this rapidly developing area.

This book, therefore, endeavours to bring together some of the dilemmas that have been encountered by practitioners who have pioneered integrated teams and suggests some possible ways forward. It is not an attempt to state the definitive line on the subject, more a wish to stimulate discussion and gather experiences from contributors who wish to challenge traditional practice. The book is written at the start of further reforms. As well as the introduction of clinical governance we are on the verge of a new system of continuing professional development to replace the credit-based postgraduate education system for general practice.[1] The Chief Medical Officer's review, based on work by Stanton and Grant, calls for a 'personal and practice development plan' to be introduced.[2,3] The stage is then set for a 'corporate' organisation to deliver primary healthcare in the community and for practice organisations to become truly inter-professional in terms of their service delivery and education. This is an opportune time therefore to take a fresh look at organisational issues in general practice.

Many questions remain unanswered:

- Are 'integrated nursing teams' a separate entity within the primary care organisation?
- What problems have been encountered?
- How can integrated nursing improve patient care?
- Will these 'teams' be a core element of future primary healthcare reforms?
- What support is required from general medical practitioners?

These questions are by no means exhaustive, but are some of the topics highlighted in the book. The contributors do not have all the answers but have tried to give an analysis of much of the early work to date.

Glyn Elwyn
June Smail
September 1998

References

1 Department of Health (1998) *A First Class Service: quality in the NHS.* DoH, London. *http://www.open.gov.uk/doh/newnhs/quality.htm*
2 Department of Health (1998) *A Review of Continuing Professional Development in Practice: a report by the Chief Medical Officer.* DoH, London. *http://www.open.gov.uk/doh/cme/cmoh.htm*
3 Stanton F and Grant J (1997) *The Effectiveness of Continuing Professional Development.* Joint Centre for Medical Education, London.

List of contributors

Jane Dauncey Director of Nursing, Oxfordshire Community Health NHS Trust

Bridgit Dimond Emeritus Professor in Law, University of Glamorgan

Glyn Elwyn Senior Lecturer and Deputy Director, Department of Postgraduate Education for General Practice and Department of General Practice, University of Wales College of Medicine

Pippa Gough Assistant Director of Nursing Policy, Royal College of Nursing, London

Kate Harris Practice Advisor for Professional Development, Primary Care Support Unit, Wiltshire Health Authority

Peter Hodder Primary Care Development Manager, Primary Health Care Service, Tile Hill, Coventry

Marcus Longley Associate Director, Welsh Institute for Health and Social Care, University of Glamorgan

Geoff Meads Professor of Health Services Development, Health Management Group, City University

John Øvretveit Professor of Health Organisation and Management, The Nordic School of Public Health

Brenda Poulton Lecturer in Nursing, School of Health Sciences, University of Ulster

Jonathan Richards General Practitioner and Visiting Professor, School of Nursing and Midwifery, University of Glamorgan

June Smail Senior Nurse for Primary Care, Gwent Health Authority and Elected Member, UKCC

Lisa Whordley Head of Primary Care Finance, Oxfordshire Community Health NHS Trust

Acknowledgements

The editors wish to thank the following people for their support and comments during the development of this book: Simon Smail, Siân Koppel, Kay Richmond, Chris Riley, Jenni Gill, Marion Evans, Nigel Stott, Steffi Williams, Peter Edwards, Howard Marsh, Melody Rhydderch and countless others in many practices who are committed to providing high quality generalist services in primary care.

Introduction

The term 'integrated teams in primary care' has been used to describe a 'team' of nurses as if they were a separate entity within the primary care organisation.[1,2] Whether having separate 'nursing teams' is a positive step is open to debate and this book provides a discussion forum for this subject. Perhaps the formation of 'nursing teams' has been a defensive reaction to the purchasing 'power' of general practitioners within fundholding and a necessary coalition to try and redress the balance where everything in the NHS within the 1990s was (or was stated to be) GP-led. Yet, despite the move to consolidate the nurses' skills, there is still one feature that allows general practitioners to remain at the centre of primary care provision – they have steadfastly, to date at least, maintained their generalist practice. Nurses and nurse educationalists, by and large, favour the route to 'specialism' and if we are to see real change in nursing practice within primary care it will be when we see the move towards a more generalist primary care nurse, albeit with special interests.

Nevertheless, general practice is changing around us, subject to relentless policy shifts, and the most recent involves an amalgamation of budgets to service a population of approximately 100 000. It will be inevitable therefore that the shape of the primary care organisation – traditionally the practice – will be transformed at the same time. Talk of a 'salaried' GP service is overheard in corridors and practices are voting with their feet to be part of primary care pilots, abandoning the Statement of Fees and Allowances, affectionately known as the 'Red Book', for the freedom to negotiate local contracts. Primary care organisations (England) and local health groups (Wales) and their equivalents in Scotland are debating what it will mean to have 'clinical governance' over local colleagues.[3,4] Nurses will want to join and be heard in these organisations.[5] As Meads suggests in the first chapter of this book, the framework which has given general practitioners both the responsibility of looking after the 'gate' to the hospital healthcare system and the control of the practice organisation is looking distinctly wobbly. It may be argued in years to come that fundholding was general practice's grand finale. Control of the financial levers will be seen as having been a mixed blessing. The 1990s spurt of GP 'power' may, with the benefit of hindsight, be seen as the crescendo of 'independent' status. A triumphant position which not only split the profession but which has also led to the current resolve to loosen the knots which have kept general practice so separate from the rest of the NHS. The speed of the un-ravelling process taking place is perhaps witness to the feeling, both within and without general practice, that there was a need for change.

Longley in Chapter 2 takes the opportunity to have a 'helicopter view' of the healthcare system. The analysis considers the position of primary healthcare services within a complex system of other changes in society and among the 'care partners' in the health service, the oft forgotten infra-structure of other (personal, social and voluntary) services, on which so much depends. The increasing speed at which technology (information exchange and other developments) are allowing a change of care location, the skill levels and in some cases the nature of the agency involved, is accelerating the move away from the traditional district hospital. This con-cept, called 'substitution', will become increasingly important as nurse triage and the nurse practitioners take on increasingly important roles in primary care organisations.[6-8]

Within this context of policy and organisational shifts, it was felt that there was a need to look critically at the concept of the 'team' in primary care. What is meant by the term and how does the widely talked about term 'integrated nursing team in primary care' fit into the wider scheme of things? The phrase 'primary healthcare team' is used relentlessly but everyone has their own view of what a primary healthcare team looks like, feels like to work in and who rightly belongs to it. Added to which is the difficulty, as Gough and Richards note in Chapter 3, that there are different ways in which 'primary healthcare' or 'primary care' as concepts are under-stood. On an international basis it can mean access to the very basics – clean water, sanitation and the provision of a rudimentary health service by unqualified personnel. In Europe the definition is usually based on direct access to mainly medical services, although this again is in a state of flux as more traditional secondary care services, such as outpatient clinics, are relocated into community-based organisations, as has happened in some fundholding practices.

In the midst of so much fluidity of definition about primary care, why have a book on integrated teams? What are they and why is there an inter-est in their development? The importance of teamwork in primary care has long been accepted. However, as the contributors to this book point out, the idea that there exists a 'team' at the heart of primary care organisations is proving to be an invalid assumption. The barriers of organisational size, task inappropriateness, role confusion, diverse accountability systems coupled with a lack of time and space has led to a gradual acceptance that the 'team' idea requires urgent reappraisal if we are to achieve a co-ordinated primary healthcare service.

Out of this realisation arose the interest in having 'practice-based nursing teams', a group more tightly bound by the aims and objectives of general practitioners (the 'owners' in many cases of the 'business'). There are many examples of such practice teams but many of the structural issues resurface. The 'team' is again ill defined and is involved in unconnected tasks. As Elwyn and Øvretveit indicate in Chapter 4, there is little evidence that enough time is devoted to meet, make decisions and provide regular feedback on performance. Frequently, each professional group perceives 'health' or 'healthcare' needs differently, often failing to communicate about individuals or groups of patients. In short, the recognised criteria for effective teamworking are absent.

Integrated nursing teams have arisen out of the realisation that teams work best if they are built around well-defined tasks, where clear leadership can be determined and agreed and where the roles of those contributing to the task are valued and well defined. The development of nursing in primary care has seen tremendous progress over the last decade, mainly within the role of the practice nurse who has been encouraged to extend the role into areas such as family planning, cervical screening, chronic disease management, prescribing and triage, as well as providing the more traditional nursing role. Alongside this new nursing practice, community nursing and health visiting have often been more conservative in their approach, although there are signs this is changing and in some areas very rapidly. Hodder describes a few of the more well-known 'integrated teams' in Chapter 7 tracing the steps that have led to their establishment and concluding that they seem to be 'sprouting up everywhere'. The next challenge will be to encourage nurses, and managers, to become involved in service planning. It is one thing to be integrated into the team protocol for asthma, and an entirely different task to contribute to the practice development plan, the local health strategy and the health purchasing agendas.[9]

Integration then in this field therefore describes the process where nurses, usually working to the list remit of a given practice, agree to form a team and appoint or nominate a leader who co-ordinates the work, resolves issues of overlap and role conflict and who is able to liaise with the medical practitioners to deliver agreed organisational objectives. In Chapter 6, Harris writes about her experience in this area and in Chapter 5, Smail brings us up-to-date with the professional training issues which nurses will face as they rise to the challenge of the primary care environment in the next millennium. The belief (based on process measures) is that integrated nursing teams are more able to provide comprehensive services to individuals, families and communities, than a disparate fragmented set of nurses working separately.[2] The effectiveness of the integrated team is related to its capability to share practice aims and responsibility for tasks and outcomes.

The financial aspect of team development is one of the most difficult areas to resolve. Whordley and Dauncey write directly about their experience in Oxford, where the Community Trust decided to develop 'self-managed' teams across the board. They point out that the funding problems for nursing in primary care are unresolved. Practice nurses are GP employees, the other nurses in primary care are Trust employees, so both camps are accountable to different systems. It is difficult to predict but it is likely that this chapter will, within a relatively short period of time perhaps, serve to record this illogical historical structure and act as a reminder to the well-recognised need to design more equitable arrangements for team member employment. Could it be, suggests Whordley, within the wit of the primary care organisations to combine the financial resources and organise unified budgets for nursing in primary care? The author succeeds in describing, even under the current strictures, an accountability framework whereby teams became entirely self-managing, to the extent that they had devolved budgets under the control of a team leader.

The Government is openly committed to a new public health and primary care agenda. Community nursing teams are now being urged to become an integral part of primary care commissioning groups, to reshape and determine services so that they are more likely to focus on peoples' and population needs. Dimond sounds a cautious note however. Teams are not legal entities and as she states in Chapter 9, 'there is no law that covers team functioning'. She discusses the difference between individual liability and team liability and emphasises the need for nurses to act within the 'scope of professional practice'. But regulatory frameworks find it difficult to capture the move to widen roles and allow increased responsibility. Integrated teams cannot fudge these issues and these areas will need clarification as pilot work encourages their implementation. Will integrated nursing teams be willing to embrace other opportunities arising from government policies? Developing integrated nursing teams is challenging, mainly due to employment and management restrictions. At present, as Poulton in Chapter 10 notes, there is little evidence to demonstrate that integrated nursing teams are more clinically and cost effective, although increased job satisfaction and role enhancement have been highlighted in a number of projects. She describes some of the evaluations that have shed light on this difficult area. But her final analysis is more to do with a sense that the structures which have evolved from the rudimentary general practice of the late 1940s into the complex primary care organisation of the 1990s cannot remain fixed on a uniprofessional model. General practitioners, with notable exceptions, have not been star team players, they are not generally renowned for anticipatory or chronic care and are slow at involving patients and consumers in shaping local services. The pressures to do all these tasks are here to stay and need addressing. This book has clear threads running through it. The team concept is suited to the delivery of discrete complex tasks that require co-ordination. A team is not a suitable model for organising large multidisciplinary organisations. Second, nurses, managers and medical practitioners should share the responsibility of both designing and delivering primary care.[10] In an evolving corporate ethos there will be a temptation to split primary care up into specialist services in the community but we would be wise not to ignore the strengths and cost effectiveness of a generalist service.[11]

References

1 Young L (1997) Improved primary care through integrated nursing. *Primary Health Care.* **7**:8–10.
2 Bull J (1998) Integrated nursing: a review of the literature. *Brit J Comm Nursing.* **3**:124–9.
3 NHS Wales (1998) *Putting Patients First.* Welsh Office, The Stationery Office, Cardiff.
4 Secretary of State for Health (1997) *The New NHS: modern, dependable.* The Stationery Office, London.
5 Young L and Poulton B (1997) Integrated nursing teams can influence locality commissioning. *Primary Health Care.* **7**:8–10.
6 Editorial (1996) Triage helps general practitioner to focus care. *Medeconomics.* **December**:53.
7 Myers PC, Lenci B and Sheldon MG (1997) A nurse practitioner as the first point of contact for urgent medical problems. *Family Practice.* **14**(5):492–7.
8 Marsh G and Dawes M (1995) Establishing a minor illness nurse in a busy general practice. *BMJ.* **310**:778–80.
9 Department of Health (1998) *A Review of Continuing Professional Development in Practice: a report by the Chief Medical Officer.* DoH, London.
10 Jones Elwyn G, Rapport FL and Kinnersley P (1998) Re-engineering the primary health care team. *Interprof Care.* **12**:189–98.
11 Royal College of General Practitioners Working Party (1996) *The Nature of General Practice.* The Royal College of General Practitioners, London.

1
The changing organisation of primary care

Geoff Meads

For the NHS, primary care is where the State and the individual meet. In its settings the dynamic of the constantly changing relationship between collective and personal responsibility for health and healthcare finds its principle expression. For the contemporary NHS, in 1998, this relationship is clearer cut than ever before – there are now simply no buffers between its central and local boundaries. Regional and Family Health Services Authorities have departed the scene and with them much of the capacity of the NHS to plan and develop itself internally. Arrangements for professional representation have undergone an apparently irrevocable process of fragmentation during the present decade, as the requirement in NHS politics for a majority consensus has been replaced by the need for simply a winning constituency to promote strategic developments, however small such constituencies might be. During the first half of the 1990s several individual general practitioner fundholders had direct access to and considerable personal influence with health ministers. Even after the change of central government in May 1997, applications by local practices to be pilots under the terms of the 1997 *NHS (Primary Care) Act* landed straight on the Secretary of State's and his ministerial colleagues' desks. From both a top-down and a bottom-up perspective the advent of alternative primary care organisations can properly be regarded as at the cutting edge of societal change. It is where the agendas of the public's elected and professional representatives come together.

Conventional general practice, of course, has long enjoyed a position of special symbolic significance in UK society. General practitioners have been in contract separately with both the individual and the State – semi-detached from both, yet still representing each to the other. The importance of this position goes back a long way. The 1911 *National Insurance Act* first associated the individual's rights to register with a general practitioner with a fundamental responsibility of the State to fund this form of primary healthcare: a form which had many of its origins in the need of an industrial island society for a fit enough labour force. Fifty per cent of would-be military recruits in 1856 had failed their medical examinations at the onset of the Crimean War, and the figures for the Boer War, four decades later, were scarcely much better. At a time when poorly resourced parish and municipal authorities on the one hand, and largely still church-based charities on the other, were both vying to establish their positions as public service organisations, and at the same time for financial reasons, restricting their responsibilities for universal care, the professional role of family doctors emerged across the country as the vehicle through which national governments could hope to guarantee the basic standards of population health. General practice supplied some sort of safety net for what then comprised the central policy of community care.[1]

A century later it is the same story. Primary care is being redefined once more in the context of public health, and its organisational forms are being addressed in ways that respond to the changing social and economic circumstances of a UK in which health policy increasingly has to encapsulate a new combination of consumerist, regional and European imperatives. The uniprofessional partnership of independent contractors has served the country well, but as the exclusive form of organisation in primary care it has now had its day. Conventional general practice is increasingly being regarded as one service outlet among many – still the focal point for healthcare in most suburbs and many market towns, but elsewhere, and especially within inner cities, the changing organisation of primary care actually means specific, individual, alternative primary care organisations increasingly hold sway.

In 1996, as Box 1.1 illustrates, most of these could be regarded as local prototypes and as such perhaps as many of these organisational initiatives could properly be expected to have a short shelf life as aspire to enduring successes. By 1998, however, what is clear is that the stage of local inventions has given way to that of national innovation. To refer now simply to the 10 000 general practices in the UK simply misses the point. The King's Fund has led the way in recognising that the new plurality is here to stay, and it can now be claimed, without being too disingenuous, that there are presently around 1000 primary care organisations in the UK.[2] As Box 1.2 illustrates, an extraordinarily large number of these are developing with national 'pilot evaluation' status. The dramatic shift from general practice to primary care is unequivocally the subject of central sponsorship. There are around 270 000 000 consultations each year in general practice. The scale and potential scope of these personal care encounters is simply too

Box 1.1 Primary care organisational developments.

Role	Purpose	Management	Population
The consortium, e.g. Isle of Wight	Effective joint planning and provision of services with health and local authorities	Steering group of individual general practice representatives, with finance and development support staff and range of GPFH/GMS allocations at individual practice levels	50 000–100 000; local community with clear boundaries
The primary care agency, e.g. Andover	Pooling of local purchaser and provider allocations to integrate and extend primary care	Executive agency under contract to local community trust and GPFHs with overall budgetary and service co-ordination responsibilities	50 000–100 000; overspill urban areas
The community development agency, e.g. East Southampton	Maximise and protect primary healthcare services contribution in local areas with significant social and economic needs	GP co-operative with multifund arrangements and shared out-of-hours rotas and information network	50 000–100 000; inner city areas; counterpart to large DGH
The community care centre, e.g. Yaxley	Provide a major unified resource for information, support and advice to exploit local potential for community self-help	Centre management group includes user representatives with strong Patients Association; integrated GPFH and SSD care management budgets and proprietary links to local residential and day care units	10 000–25 000; small towns, suburbs with single large established general practices

Source: Meads G (1996) Future options for general practice. *British Journal of Health Care Management,* **2**(7):372–4.

Box 1.2 Let a thousand flowers bloom. Emerging organisations in primary care – Spring 1998 (Best estimates in rounded figures).

- 100 Primary medical services pilots*

- 40 GP commissioning group pilots*

- 350 Locality commissioning groups*

- 30 Resource centres

- 10 Health parks

- 30 Consortia

- 10 Primary care group (trust) pilots*

- 60 Total purchasing pilots*

- 10 Health action zones*

- 30 Community care centres

- 20 Health CALL/BUPA (etc) primary care centres

- 10 Hospital trust primary care units

- 10 Pastoral care centres

- 50 Centres for complementary therapies

- 30 Healthy living centres*

- Plus GPFH models

* Indicates those schemes directly subject, fully or in part, to centrally arranged evaluations.

Sources: Singer R (1997) *GP Commissioning: an inevitable evolution.* Radcliffe Medical Press, Oxford; Mays N (1997) *Total Purchasing Pilots Evaluation: interim report.* King's Fund, London; Mays N and Dixon J (1996) *Purchasing Plurality in UK Health Care.* King's Fund, London; Peckham S, Macdonald J and Taylor P (1996) *Primary Care and Public Health.* The Public Health Trust, Birmingham; Meads G (ed) (1995), *Future Options for General Practice.* Radcliffe Medical Press, Oxford; Internal and External NHS communications including, for example, NHSE (July 1997) *Personal Medical Services under the NHS (Primary Care) Act 1997: a guide to local evaluation* and NHSE (October 1997) *Health Action Zones: invitation to bid.* EL(97)65.

enormous for any government to ignore. It would do so at its peril. Contemporary primary care has to be organised in ways that, at worst, do not limit tomorrow's political imperatives and, at best, actually promote the changing balance of responsibilities between the modern State and its individual citizens.

The local ownership of an efficient, effective, equitable nationwide health system – this is the policy ideal and the prize in which integrated teams including nurses may in the future share. Indeed, as managers diminish, as cost pressures further promote substitution and the majority of general practitioners revert to their physician roots, nurses could do even better. The viability of future primary care organisations and the capacity of community nurses to develop as successful leaders of new local team partnerships are arguably one and the same thing. But just as primary care organisations will have no standard models, neither will the community-based nursing profession of the future. Integrated teams could well represent a glittering prize for nurses, but there will inevitably, in terms of traditional rights and status, be some penalties to pay and sacrifices to endure as well.

References

1   A succinct explanation of the role of primary healthcare in the history of the pre- and post-1948 health service nationally is provided in Levitt R, Wall A and Appleby J (1995) *The Reorganised NHS* (5th ed). Chapman and Hall, London. For a more profound insight, Sir George Godber's masterly Heath Clark Lecture remains invaluable – Godber G (1973) *The Health Service: past, present and future*. Athlone Press, London.
2   Mays N and Dixon J (1996) *Purchasing Plurality in UK Health Care*. King's Fund, London.

Further reading

Secretary of State for Health (1997) *The New NHS: modern, dependable*. The Stationery Office, London (Chapter 5).
Bagnall P and Gardner L (1997) Primary care nursing: managing the journey ahead. *Primary Care*. 7(6):2–7.
House of Commons Select (Health) Committee (1993) *Changing Childbirth*. HMSO, London.
NHS Executive (1996) *Nurse Practitioner Evaluation Project*. Department of Health, London.
Meads G (1996) All together. *Nursing Standard*. II(7):16.

2
Integrated nursing teams and healthcare 'substitution'

Marcus Longley

It often seems that there is only one certain thing about the future of healthcare – that there is *nothing* certain about the future of healthcare. This chapter sets the debate about integrated nursing teams in the context of this changing scene and addresses the question, 'Do such teams go with the flow of other change, or do they cut across it?' It uses the concept of 'substitution' as an analytical framework.

The changing world

Because of the extent and complexity of the factors influencing the future of healthcare, a degree of simplification is required in their examination. Some of the key issues, of particular relevance to primary/community nursing, are considered here under three broad headings:

- changes in the wider NHS
- changes on the borders of the NHS (with 'care partners' such as individuals looking after themselves, social care agencies and the private sector)
- changes in society.

All of these are to some extent interrelated and all impinge on integrated nursing in the community (*see* Figure 2.1).

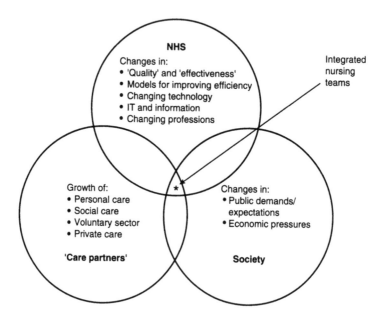

Figure 2.1 Integrated nursing at the centre of change.

Changing society

When considering broader changes in society a whole host of issues is relevant, but two are perhaps of particular importance. Public demands and expectations of welfare services generally – and of healthcare in particular – are changing. The development of 'Charters' covering most aspects of public service provision is both an expression of, and a stimulant to, an increasing view that public services are there to serve the public, and that the public are their 'customers' with a set of legitimate expectations in relation to service standards. It is perhaps significant that the post-1997 Labour Government willingly accepted the notion of Charters and continued their development and refinement – 'consumerism' is no longer a partisan issue.

Economic pressures on government expenditure have an even longer ancestry and are recognised and accepted by British governments of every hue. There will therefore always be a background pressure to control costs. This is given added impetus by somewhat alarmist projections of the cost implications for the future of an aging population, although the UK is better placed than most developed countries to cope with this change.[1] Different approaches to this problem have been explored: imposing time costs (waiting lists), dilution of service (reducing the 'intensity' of care by providing fewer tests and drugs), reducing length of stay, adopting a more cost-conscious approach to quality (minimum rather than optimum standards), explicit rationing,[2] and even *de facto* privatisation of services (such as general dental services). Many will continue to feature in future policy developments.

The changing NHS

Within the NHS, successive governments have prioritised the issues of 'quality' and 'effectiveness' in healthcare.[3] Despite the complexities of definition of both these terms they have considerable currency, even if only because it is impossible to argue that quality and effectiveness are not important! The attractiveness for politicians is clear – people suffer from poor care and it wastes money.

Governments in the 1980s and 1990s in the UK have also flirted with new models for improving efficiency within healthcare,[4] moving from a collectivist approach where healthcare recognised few internal divisions other than the decades-old split between general practitioners and specialists, to a radical attempt to create within the NHS a multiplicity of providers and purchasers, to the 'New Labour' synthesis where the term 'modernisation' is used to convey the impression of integration and partnership, but where the internal market is retained in all but name. Each change was in part at least designed to improve efficiency and the lack of realistic estimates of costs within the Labour-proposed reforms would suggest that further experimentation with new 'more efficient' models is still likely.[5] Certainly, the influence of primary care (and general practitioners in particular) on the shape of service provision increased significantly with the advent of general practitioner fundholding and commissioning, and looks set to continue in this high profile role under the Labour Government.

Changes in healthcare technology represent a powerful force for change, covering developments from the 'hard' end – new equipment, drugs, diagnostic tests, surgical procedures – to the 'soft' end – ways of providing care and the organisation of services consequent upon such changes.[6] Such developments are not new, of course, although there is every reason to believe that the pace of change is set to quicken in the coming years, particularly as the impact of a better understanding of the genetic determinants of health leads to a new panoply of tests and therapies.[7]

One important development is the exponential growth in the means of gathering together and processing data – information technology (IT) – and the resulting information.[8] This will manifest itself in four main ways. First, the use of 'smart cards' and greater use of electronic data interchange will provide more *information about patients*, in a form which is easily portable (of particular relevance to community staff) and which has the potential to bring together separate sets of data, all under the patient's own control. Second, there will be available an unimaginable ocean of *information for patients*, about all conceivable aspects of health and healthcare, for all those who are interested and who have the access and skills to tap into the worldwide web and other sources. Healthcare professionals will increasingly be dealing with patients who may know more about certain aspects of their treatment than the professional, and may similarly be seriously *mis*informed too. These 'information rich' patients will demand more of the professionals' time (to explain, justify and correct misunderstandings) and will challenge any remaining notions of passivity and subservience in the patient role. Third, there will be more *information on effectiveness* as the drive towards evidence-based practice continues, and IT makes it readily available to all professionals, hopefully in a form which complements their practice. Finally, there may even be more *information on efficiency*, as cost-benefit and cost-effectiveness data is generated in ever greater quantities and disseminated more effectively to decision makers.

Partly in response to this change, and partly in an attempt to realise their own goals, the healthcare professions are also undergoing a period of substantial change. Many patients still believe – and want to believe – that the 'doctor knows best'. On the other hand, they are increasingly coming to challenge such notions,[9] as popular belief in the ability of science and medicine to control risk is questioned.[10] The privileged position of the professions as self-regulating and legally-protected groups has been based on two foundations: a belief in their competence and in their commitment – they know what they are doing and they act in the best interests of their clients. Both of these are beliefs under attack.[11] Governments are considering whether the professional agenda contradicts the Government's own interest in promoting efficiency and quality. The public, in part encouraged by Government pronouncements and Charters, and in part by using the courts, increasingly challenges the power of individual professionals. There has been some inter-professional rivalry in public, over issues such as the nurse's extended role and competence to prescribe and dissenting voices have also emerged within professions, such as the obstetricians who have lauded the woman's right to control her care, and professional leaders who have publicly admitted that some of their fellow doctors and nurses are not providing good care. Witness the events surrounding the Bristol case in 1998. The net effect of this is to undermine the professional 'mystery' traditionally attached to doctors and others,[12] and also the relative autonomy of the professions as organised labour, and of individual professionals in their clinical practice.

Changing 'care partners'

There is also a set of important changes taking place among those with whom the NHS works to deliver care – notably the social services, voluntary and private sectors. The exhortations to work more closely with partners in social services become stronger with each new government, and the pressure to find new ways of working with the voluntary sector and with private service providers and financiers is also likely to continue. Joint funding remains, though, a difficult arrangement to negotiate, as one apocryphal definition of the term illustrates: 'It requires two people to share one kitty, when one is drinking triple single malts and the other diet cokes.'

Patients themselves are also being drawn more into the net, with explicit attempts by Government to specify the responsibilities of service users in Charters, and to provide support for those who agree to care for their dependent relatives, as well as emphasising personal responsibility in other areas of welfare provision such as pensions.

The impact on healthcare: substitution

All of these 'guesses' about the future could, of course, be wrong in terms of timing or extent. There is a general consensus, though, that development in these *directions* is almost inevitable. That is not to presume a determinist position – that it is bound to happen and therefore there is nothing we can do about it – but rather to show the direction in which change is nudging healthcare, and to highlight the opportunities for those with their own vision of future best practice. If integrated nursing care moves with the flow of these changes, then its progress is likely to be more rapid and longer lasting.

The difficulty in this sort of analysis, though, lies primarily in bringing the various strands together, and in imagining their *combined* impact on the pattern of healthcare. One approach to this is to use the framework offered by the concept of substitution,[13] which provides one way of systematically identifying the possible organisational consequences of change in the future.[14]

The pattern of healthcare provision in the UK has been dominated by the central role of the district general hospital (DGH) since the early 1960s,[15] almost regardless of the several attempts to reform the administrative structure which periodically raged around it. Care was overwhelmingly provided in four types of locality:

- the patient's own home
- the GP's surgery/health centre
- the district general hospital
- the teaching or other specialist hospital (*see* Figure 2.2).

Towards the end of this period, however, the gathering strength of the forces for change outlined above began to have an appreciable effect on this hitherto stable structure. For ease of analysis, four types of impact – or 'substitution' – can be discerned.

First, substitution of *location* occurs when services are moved from one place to another, but stay substantially unaltered in the process. One example is the relocation of outpatient consultation clinics from hospital to general practitioner's surgery. Although a number of benefits are claimed from such moves, the service is usually still provided by a secondary care doctor to whom patients are referred by the general practitioner, and the range of examinations is very similar.

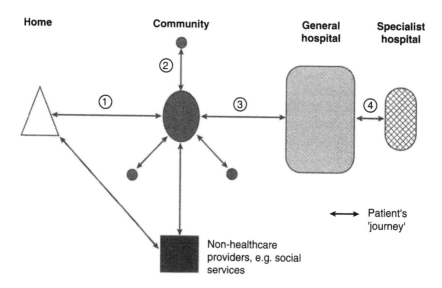

Figure 2.2 Healthcare – now.

Second, there are substitutions of *technology*, where patients are diagnosed or treated in quite different ways as the result of the adoption of a new technology. Perhaps the most obvious example is the change in the treatment of stomach ulcers, where surgical procedures were common until the advent of suitable drug therapies. The impending developments stemming from the new genetics could herald the biggest wave of technological substitution yet seen in healthcare.

Third, there are *staff* substitutions, where the same task is performed by different members of staff. Within primary care there are many examples of such substitution, some of them associated with the major growth in the number of practice nurses, a proportion of whose work consists of tasks previously undertaken by general practitioners. Within hospitals, the role of the junior doctor has for some time attracted critical attention – for example, one study estimated that between 15% and 22% of junior doctors' time on wards involved activities which could be carried out by other staff.[16]

Finally, there have been some examples of substitution of *agency*, where, for example, social services or the voluntary sector have assumed responsibility – either *de facto* or *de jure* – from the NHS and *vice versa*, or responsibility has explicitly been shared. The continuing emphasis on local interagency collaboration and the development of 'seamless' care is likely further to fuel this sort of substitution.

Of course, many developments in practice illustrate more than one type of substitution. For example, change of location can actually lead to very different ways of providing the service and different use of technology, or technological change, opens the possibility for the use of different staff, and so on.

The net impact of these changes has been gradually to loosen the structure initiated by the creation of DGHs and other developments, and sometimes to question the rationale for certain elements of service organisation. Figure 2.3 illustrates in simplified, diagrammatic form some of the changes which are taking place. A gradually increasing range of services previously available only in hospital (such as post-operative care for day patients or kidney dialysis) is now available in the home, and telemedicine will further enhance the possibilities for domiciliary care. At the home/community interface ① patients are increasingly making choices about the services they require, looking to complementary medicine, community pharmacy and the voluntary sector, as well as general practitioner-centred care. The services immediately available to the general practitioner ② have expanded considerably in recent years, partly because entirely new services have been developed, and partly through various substitutions – of nurses and others for GPs, and through locational substitution of various hospital services. New combinations of services are emerging at the interface of community and secondary healthcare and social services ③.

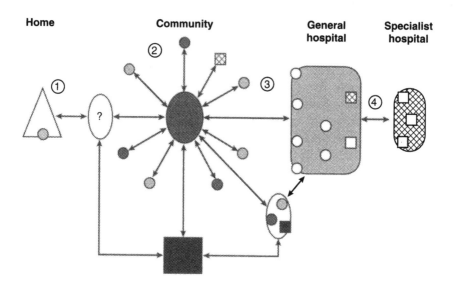

Figure 2.3 Healthcare – future.

Examples range from new uses for community hospitals embracing all agencies, to open-access arrangements for general practitioners to secondary care services. Finally, the balance of services between secondary and specialised healthcare is shifting, with some elements becoming more widely available in DGHs (such as the significant expansion in cardiology services), and others moving in the opposite direction (for example, cancer services under the influence of the Calman-Hine review).

Change on this scale eventually calls into question the continuing rationale for the pattern of services illustrated in Figure 2.2. For example, how long can the general practitioner be expected adequately to co-ordinate an ever-growing complexity of services in the community, and how much does the DGH have to lose before it ceases to be viable? The time may be fast approaching for a radical review of this pattern.

The impact of substitution on primary care and community nursing

What impact has this series of changes, or substitutions, had on nursing in the primary care and community settings?

Perhaps the most obvious impact has been primarily a locational substitution – the transfer of elements of care from hospital to the community setting. There have been substantial reductions in inpatient lengths of stay, partly as a result of the growth of day surgery and other developments at the hospital end, and partly because of the greater capacity and willingness of primary care to undertake procedures previously reserved for secondary care. As a result, over the period 1959–90, the number of non-psychiatric beds in England fell by 45%. GPs and nurses are now having to assume responsibility for elements of post-operative care, for example, which previously would have been carried out by their hospital colleagues.

Closely related to this has been an element of increasing sophistication in the type of care provided in primary settings – a technological substitution. This is manifest both in the care provided to earlier hospital discharges and also to those patients now wholly treated in the community.

Not surprisingly, staff roles have also changed substantially. This has been achieved partly through the development of new categories of staff – the practice nurse emerged rapidly from a very limited base during the early 1990s – but more often by existing staff adapting to changed circumstances. General practitioners are now providing a number of services previously the responsibility of secondary care, as are their nursing colleagues. The development of roles has not been an entirely passive phenomenon, of course, as many staff have actively sought new, more demanding roles, and the education and training to carry them out.

Substitution of funding responsibility has been most obvious in the area of continuing care. There has been a substantial growth in private sector provision of nursing home beds, and changes in the acute sector of healthcare have often forced social services departments to modify their own priorities to cope with the increasing numbers of older patients being discharged from the NHS.

If one puts together these various changes, it is possible to see that the future of primary care will increasingly be characterised by greater *autonomy* and *accountability* – the higher levels of skilled care and raised expectations, together with the sheer pressure of workload, will demand that primary care nurses operate with greater autonomy, more along the lines of the midwife rather than the first generation of practice nurses. This will have to be balanced by clear and appropriate lines of accountability, a difficult proposition given the somewhat fragmented nature of much of primary care, where there are often no natural groupings of nurses to support and monitor each other's practice. The managerial form which this will engender will be localised *contracts with practices* rather than GPs – this is already evident in the recent NHS White Paper,[5] where the planning role of nurses is specifically mentioned in relation to primary care groups. This will develop alongside improved *quality monitoring* of all professional staff, perhaps through the development of accreditation within the broad ambit of 'clinical governance', as well as more sophisticated *risk management* through more protocols, backed up by clinical audit.

Primary care will offer an *increased range of provision* of clinical services, involving all members of the primary healthcare team. Pressures – both internally and externally generated – for *value for money* at all levels will continue. There will even perhaps be an increased emphasis on *'management'* within practices, including the development of a 'corporate focus' for teams which increasingly see themselves as different from other groups of local providers.

Where do integrated nursing teams fit in?

The net result of the changes described in this chapter is to change both the *quantity* and the *quality* of primary healthcare. In short, primary care professionals in the future will be doing more and doing it differently. To the extent that processes of substitution are changing the nature of primary care, therefore, any attempt to reformulate working practices and philosophies to meet such changing demands is to be welcomed.

The time for change is ripe, but are integrated nursing teams the right sort of change? The substitution framework offers one way to evaluate the appropriateness of any proposed organisational change such as integrated nursing teams in the changing context of healthcare. Four key questions are set out in Box 2.1.

Box 2.1   Criteria for assessing the appropriateness of organisational change in the context of substitution.

Substitution	Key question: Does the organisational change ...
1 Location	allow the development of new services in the locality in the future?
2 Technology	allow for increasing specialisation within the organisation?
3 Staff	allow for flexibility of roles?
4 Agency	help bridge interagency barriers?

The reality of integrated nursing teams, to the extent that they have developed to date, is discussed elsewhere in this book. But *in theory* they should be particularly well adapted to cope with substitutions of *staff* and *technology*. In these areas, the future will be characterised by frequently changing roles, in part stimulated by new technological capacities, and in part by professionals' desire to adapt the services they provide to better meet the needs (and changing needs) of their clients. This will call for elements of increased specialisation within the teams and also flexibility. It might be argued that one of the prime arguments for integrated nursing teams is that they offer just these characteristics.

As far as substitutions of *location* are concerned, integrated nursing teams clearly have some advantages. To the extent that the teamworking increases the motivation, skills and efficiency of team members, then the capacity to absorb new services increases. However, many other factors are also relevant here, particularly the resource elements of revenue and capital. The pressures on all parts of primary care have increased significantly since the advent of the general practice contract and other developments of the 1990s, and increased efficiency can only go part of the way to bridging the gap between supply and demand. Capital availability often proves to be a particularly inflexible element in this balancing act. Capital resources (including IT and major equipment, as well as buildings) have historically been heavily concentrated in secondary care, with comparatively little scope for attracting new resources to primary care. Locational substitution, therefore, usually has to be accompanied by transference of capital resources from the hospital to the clinic or surgery setting, a process more easy to contemplate than realise. Integrated nursing teams can achieve much in terms of efficiency, but large scale movement of resources may require other initiatives, and the intent of the recent White Papers may help.[5,17]

Perhaps the weakest element in this analysis relates to the capacity of integrated nursing teams to address the need for closer interagency working, especially in the links between primary healthcare and social services. There would appear to be little to offer social workers and others in teams which are specifically designed to strengthen the links between nurses. It might be argued that integrated nursing teams are but the first step towards greater interagency working and that it is important that nurses first resolve their own internal links, before looking to form closer alliances with others. This may prove to be true. However, the history of poor collaboration between health and local government services indicates the size of the challenge remaining.

Conclusion

Integrated nursing teams will not solve all the problems of primary care. What they can do is provide a way of working that is in many respects in tune with broader developments in healthcare, and which is well adapted to meet future changes. One major potential flaw is in the exclusive focus on links within nursing, which may be to the exclusion of better links with other professionals providing services to the very same patients/clients.

References

1 Organisation for Economic Cooperation and Development (1995) *Economic Outlook*. OECD, Paris.
2 Klein R (1994) Can we restrict the health care menu? *Health Policy.* **27**(2):104–5.
3 Ranade W (1994) *A Future for the NHS? Healthcare in the 1990s.* Longman, London.
4 Timmins N (1996) *The Five Giants: a biography of the welfare state.* Fontana Press, London.
5 Secretary of State for Health (1997) *The New NHS: modern, dependable.* The Stationery Office, London.
6 Avery J (1995) *Future Trends in technology.* World Health Organisation, Copenhagen.
7 Longley MJ (1997) Assessing the new genetics (editorial). *Brit J Health Care Management.* **3**(3):124.
8 Engelbrecht R (1995) *Information Society.* World Health Organisation, Copenhagen.
9 Williams SJ and Calnan M (1996) The 'limits' of medicalisation?: modern medicine and the lay populace in 'late' modernity. *Soc Sci Med.* **42**(12):1609–20.
10 Gabe J (ed) (1995) *Medicine, Health and Risk: sociological approaches.* Blackwell, Oxford.
11 Gabe J, Kelleher D and Williams G (eds) (1995) *Challenging Medicine.* Routledge, London.
12 Johnson TJ (1972) *Professions and Power.* Macmillan, London.
13 Warner M (1991) Health strategy for the 1990s: five areas for substitution. In: A Harrison and S Bruscini (eds) *Health Care UK 1991: an annual review of health care policy.* King's Fund Institute, London.
14 Longley MJ and Warner M (1995) Future health scenarios: strategic issues for the British health service. *Long Range Planning.* **28**(4):22–32.

15 Minister of Health (1962) *A Hospital Plan for England and Wales.* Cmnd 1604, HMSO, London.

16 Greenhalgh T (1994) *The Interface Between Junior Doctors and Nurses: a research study for the DoH. Final Report.* Unpublished.

17 Secretary of State for Wales (1998) *Putting Patients First: NHS Cymru Wales.* Welsh Office, Cardiff.

3
The political and policy context

Pippa Gough and Jonathan Richards

'If millions of nurses in a thousand different places articulate the same ideas and convictions about primary healthcare and come together as one force, then they could act as a powerhouse for change. I believe such a change is coming and that nurses around the globe whose work touches us intimately, will greatly help to bring it about.'[1]

Introduction

Numerous chapters in this book rehearse the failings of the so-called primary healthcare team (PHCT) as a prelude to further examination of the integrated nursing team (INT). The PHCT organisationally and structurally has been too big, roles have been poorly defined, traditional hierarchies have gone largely unchallenged, interprofessional liaison has been undeveloped, accountability systems have been too diverse and objectives rarely negotiated or shared. The argument then follows that the INT has evolved primarily as result of this failure. INTs are structurally the right size, leadership is clearly determined, individual contribution is valued and recognised, lines of communication are good, individual and team autonomy is pronounced and above all the doctor–nurse power dynamic is not an immediate issue.

Most nurses with experience of working within primary healthcare over the last decade would recognise and relate strongly to the above critique and would agree that the INT is appealing as a progressive way forward – particularly when viewed in the context of the changes in health and social care and societal expectation and demand described in Chapter 2.

These may not be the only factors, however, that explain the growing popularity of INTs and why they seem so 'right' for the moment. Consideration should also be given to the INT as the vehicle for enabling nurses to redefine primary healthcare in its broadest sense, i.e. in a way that allows the breadth of the nursing contribution to primary healthcare to find expression. In other words, is the INT simply a reorganisation of established professionals with stable roles into teams for management purposes, or a reassertion of a way of thinking, acting and being for nurses working within primary health care?

INTs and primary healthcare: redefining the concept

In the Introduction, Elwyn and Smail allude to the conceptual confusion that exists over the term 'primary healthcare' and the way it has been used within the policy arena. Within the Alma Ata definition,[2] primary healthcare is about a focus on health rather than illness; an orientation to health care delivery that is about accessibility (providing care where people are – their homes, their workplaces and their schools); equity; multi-sectoral collaboration; breadth rather than depth; community involvement, motivation and participation; and partnerships, not only with individuals but with families, groups and communities.

Within the UK the term 'primary healthcare' whilst unendingly trendy, has also become a somewhat meaningless catch all. It is frequently used to describe not only the breadth of activities set out above but also something far less broad and more tightly focused on the delivery of secondary care services within community settings. Conceptually and pragmatically the two are at opposite ends of the spectrum. One starts from the position of wellness and the maintenance of health within communities, usually outwith the medical domain; the other is about treating illness outside of institutions. Both are valuable activities to pursue but they are not the same thing. Each requires different approaches, knowledge and skills. Neither does one subsume the other, nor do they exist in a hierarchical relationship of importance and value. Ideally, both can and should be offered as part of a whole service – but how often is this truly the case?

In 1986, Vuori suggested that:[3]

> 'The claim that primary medical care is identical with primary healthcare is particularly dear to those health authorities and health professionals who want to give the impression of being all for primary healthcare but who in fact are either opposed to it or have not quite understood what it means. It is easy to refer to the activities of the primary care physicians ... equate them with primary healthcare and then proceed to say that no further development of primary healthcare is needed.'

One of the major political issues in the development of primary healthcare, and the role of nurses within this, over the last decade has been the decision by the last Government to place the lead for primary care with general medical practitioners. The rhetoric of the 'primary care-led NHS' (and note here the loss of the word 'health') is predicated upon an interesting conceptual sleight of hand that suggests primary healthcare is in fact synonymous with primary medical care or general practice. *The Primary Care Act 1996* is the prize example here in terms of misnomer, centred as it is on setting up pilot sites to test out new ways of delivering not the breadth of primary healthcare but rather personal and general medical services.

This is not purely a matter of semantics or sloppy shorthand. Rather it can be argued that this in fact denotes a determined policy shift to realign the NHS, and the use of scarce resources, on the treatment of ill health and disease. This in turn allows the costs of health maintenance and the response to health need to be shunted on to other services and Government departments.

General practice tends to be focused on individualistic, episodic, 'come and get it' treatment for symptoms of disease, with some health education and health maintenance activities in the form of individual screening offered on the periphery. In short, general practice, quite rightly, provides a service to meet *healthcare*, rather than *health needs*. This is not to be critical – there have been some exceptional developments in general practice over the last 10 years, many to the benefit of the development of nurses and nursing within that context. However, general practice can never be the whole of primary healthcare – it is but one dimension of it – and primary healthcare nursing outside of general practice has struggled to find expression. This is especially in relation to those activities centred on well populations, community development, public health approaches and the notion of social support. These have been relegated to the margins of the new primary care-led NHS. The insidious 'disinvestment' in health visiting and school nursing over the last few years is a prime example of this policy approach.

On the other hand, for those nurses, such as practice nurses and nurse practitioners, whose roles centre on general practice and the practice population, this has been a time of their ascendancy with dramatic effects on the breadth of quality services that general practice patients now receive.

The resynthesising and integration of primary healthcare nursing expertise and practice into one team would seem to be a timely political and pragmatic response to these issues.

The professional and labour market context

The current healthcare environment, and within this primary healthcare, is characterised by rapid change, ongoing fiscal constraints, shifting professional boundaries and more complex healthcare needs requiring equally complex responses. Healthcare reforms of the last decade have resulted in myriad changes to both form and function of the health services and all of these factors have prompted the search for new ways of configuring the healthcare workforce and more effective and economic methods of care delivery. Skill-mix reviews, reprofiling and re-engineering exercises and the examination of the efficacy of a multiskilled and 'generic' healthcare workforce are some of the responses.[4,5] Many of these centre on the nursing workforce.

The healthcare professions are often accused of being rigidly tribal, inflexible and unresponsive to change and the basic premise of many of these initiatives is that nurses, in particular, can be replaced by other staff (assistive personnel) who are drawn from the local labour market, can be trained more quickly and more cheaply and will work more flexibly and for lower wages. Many of these analyses have presented nursing as a series of disaggregated tasks, the component parts of which can be carried out by non-professional personnel at less cost.

At core, these ideas about labour utilisation are always advanced on the basis of being in the patient's interests; the proposed new models are 'patient centred' or 'patient focused'. Often attempts to modify these approaches are seen as motivated by professional self-interest, tribalism and intransigence. Whilst such motives undoubtedly exist in some instances, professional commitment to expertise and quality in the face of 'dumbing down' is almost never viewed as professional commitment.

The challenge for nursing is to be able to embrace the thinking behind skill-mix and multiskilling but to demonstrate these concepts as skill-sharing, i.e. the non-hierarchical development of skills at the boundaries of nursing practice. This relates to expansion of role in line with the Code of Professional Conduct and the principles set out in the Scope of Professional Practice and does not detract from a clear professional identity and core skills.[6,7] Skill-sharing in this sense is premised upon good teamworking and enhances continuity of care and cohesion of services to the patient.

INTs offer a way in which the concepts of professional integration and integrated care, premised upon the notion of skill-sharing and the development of a mix of individuals with a range of skills rather than skill-mixing or multiskilling to the lowest common denominator, can be demonstrated. As such, the INTs that are emerging currently are the model for quality and expert nursing across the board of healthcare in the future.

McWhinney, writing for the medical profession, reviews the history of family medicine and comments:[8]

> 'Two lessons we would do well to ponder:
> 1 If the profession is failing to meet a public need, society will find some way of meeting the need, if necessary by turning to a group outside of the profession.
>
> 2 Professions evolve in response to social pressures, sometimes in ways that conflict with the expressed intentions of their members.'

It would seem crazy to create an alternative workforce to nursing purely because nurses were not being enabled to make the contribution, particularly within primary healthcare, for which they have the potential. Individuals respond to change, or threat of change, in different ways. Some feel more comfortable with certainties of their established roles and relationships. Others, such as those who are spearheading the INT movement, will relish the challenges of developing the future for themselves and their patients.

Further encouragement for adaptation and change came from the Chief Nursing Officers of the four Health Departments of the UK who instituted the 'Heathrow Debate' in 1994. The ensuing report summarised the challenges facing the profession and suggested that:[9]

> 'In response to these challenges nurses cannot rest on their laurels. They must monitor how attitudes are changing and consider the implications. Then, building on existing roles, they must take on an active role, moving out to educate the public in all its guises to broaden the understanding of the nature of nursing and enable the expression of nursing through other roles.'

The new NHS

INTs reflect many of the themes and expectations contained within the White Papers for Wales, Scotland and England which set out the Government's vision for the NHS over the next 10 years.[10–12] This new policy direction has, within the text, intention and pages of the papers at least, created significant opportunities not only for nurses generally but for community nurses in particular.

Key themes within the policy changes are those of collaboration, partnership and integration, quality and effectiveness. The vision reflects many of the tenets of the 'third way' which underpins the policies of the new political regime. That is, it rejects the command and control model of welfarism of the 1970s but also steers away from the notion of the free market approach and the vagaries of the internal market with all its attendant fragmentation and bureaucracy. It maintains the separation between purchasing and provision, continues to promote and build on the importance of primary care, but within this aims to dismantle GP fundholding, and keeps a decentralised responsibility for management and the use of resources. Central control is reconfigured in the guise of statutory penalties on organisations for failure to hit quality expectations and the internal market, based upon the harsh demands of the contract culture, is replaced with a new system of integrated care based on partnerships and service agreements. Finally, technology and use of information is highlighted as being key to the spread of good practice.

The concept of 'clinical governance' is introduced as a key way of promoting professional responsibility for quality of care. Although this concept has yet to be defined in detail or in terms of concrete policy, clinical governance should be premised upon the notion of systems of peer review within environments of support, trust and respect, good teamworking, allocation of space and time for clinicians and teams to reflect upon practice, and enhanced professional autonomy. This in turn feeds into the concept of professional self-regulation in its purest sense, wherein professionals feel empowered and enabled to make difficult decisions in the management of risk.

It can be argued that INTs, in terms of approach, structure and philosophy, have been ahead of their time in that they reflect absolutely the major underpinning tenets of the White Papers and provide an excellent model for implementing many of the new policy requirements within the primary healthcare context. In this respect their importance cannot be underestimated.

As well as setting out new mechanisms for quality and efficiency, the White Papers also set out new structural arrangements for commissioning health services in the future. The focus for these new arrangements centre on primary healthcare and the dismantling of GP fundholding as the main mechanism for purchasing and providing primary and some secondary care services. In the future, commissioning at a local level will be undertaken by new bodies, primary care groups (PCGs) in England and Wales, with a responsibility for commissioning primary care services, in line with the health authorities Health Improvement Plan, for localities of about 100 000 head of population. It is stipulated clearly in the White Papers that nurses are to be key stakeholders and players within these new arrangements.[11,12]

Issues of marginalisation and involvement

Many commentators upon the present state of the NHS have used the phrase coined during the cultural revolution in China, 'Let a thousand flowers bloom!' The White Papers make much of flexibility and the need for services to be commissioned to fit the context into which they will be placed.[10-12] There will be a large number of stakeholders wishing to ensure that the flowers that bloom are the ones that suit their particular tastes and sensibilities. For nurses, the challenge is to ensure that their voices will be heard. There is no doubt that, because of the lead they have had over the last decade for developing primary care services, many general practitioners have assumed that it is they who will be leading the development of PCGs and the new commissioning arrangements within the new structures. Anecdotal information at the time of writing suggests that GPs have already leapt into action to secure their position at the helm, with very little thought being given as to how nurses and other healthcare professionals can be involved in the process. This is despite continued reminders from the Government on a variety of public platforms that community nurses must be part of the new arrangements.

A number of factors militate against nurses finding their place at the policy high tables in this respect. Nurses do not have the ready made infrastructure that allows them to organise and network in order to develop a strategy for involvement and action. Nurses working in the community and in general practice do not have a Local Nursing Committee, as doctors do their Local Medical Committee. Neither have nurses been part of the loose alliances of GP fundholders or commissioning GPs or multifunds that have developed over the past decade and which are now acting as efficient channels of communication and planning for the new arrangements. Within existing structures, nurses have not been invited to form commissioning groups or purchasing pilots. Although some innovative projects have included nurses on the management board and some nursing teams and individuals have developed small local projects, in the main nurses are still viewed as the handmaidens in the corridors of power in most localities and districts.

Whereas serving general practitioners are represented at every level of decision making in most localities and health authorities, the community and practice nurse voice is not heard on many committees. On those bodies where a nurse is invited, the nurse is usually a nurse manager with a management agenda to pursue, rather than primarily a clinical one.

Finally, because of a legacy of medical domination, however benevolent, and a recent history of nurses being the employees of medical practitioners within primary care, many nurses appear to be waiting to be invited on to PCGs once they have already been formulated and set up by the GPs in their area. If PCGs are to benefit from the contribution of nurses, then nurses need to be involved from the start of the discussions and planning, not co-opted in once the blueprint has been drawn up and agreed.

INTs offer a wealth of experience and knowledge appropriate to the new locality commissioning arrangements. They have for many years been developing a service premised upon a broad definition of primary health-care. They are knowledgeable about health need and healthcare need assessment and are used to commissioning against this assessment. Nurses within INTs know the local area, the services and approaches that work and are appropriate, and what will be rejected or accepted by local communities. They are used to providing a service that helps local communities to maximise their health as well as to enabling access to services that will ensure illnesses are treated efficiently and effectively. If PCGs are charged with commissioning in order to develop primary healthcare, rather than simply primary medical care, then the lack of INT involvement in the new arrangements will be a damaging omission. Commissioning built around the skills of approaches developed within INTs will provide a robust and valuable model for the rest of the country to follow.

The new public health

Much emphasis has been placed by the new political regime on the social context of health and the impact on health of poverty and social exclusion. Two Green Papers have been published in England and Scotland setting out the Government's policy intentions in respect of creating a healthier nation.[13,14] Community nurses, particularly where they are working in integrated community nursing teams, are a key workforce in delivering this new public health agenda. Nurses, in particular INTs working to a robust health needs assessment, are already working across agency boundaries as well as across the wellness/illness spectrum; they offer an important point of access to most healthcare services; they employ community development and public approaches as well as individual interventions; and they operate in all of the key settings listed in the White Papers, namely neighbourhoods, schools and workplaces.

Conclusion

The emerging political and policy agendas of the current Government provide a fitting backdrop for the continued development of the integrated nursing team. In order to take their rightful place within the new arrangements, nurses involved in this new way of working must meet the challenges offered and grasp the new opportunities as they emerge. Through past, and sometimes bitter, experience we know that this will not always take place within an environment of encouragement and support. Nurses can no longer afford to wait in the wings to be invited to join the other players on centre stage. A new script is waiting to be written and this time, through the example and power of the pioneering INTs, nurses can at last be among the authors.

References

1 Mahler H (1988) World Health: 2000 and beyond (address by Director General, WHO). *World Hospitals.* **24**(1):32–7.
2 World Health Organisation (1978) *Report on the Primary Health Care Conference*, Alma Ata. WHO, Geneva.
3 Vuori H (1986) Health for all: primary health care and general practitioners. *JRCGP.* **36**:398–402.
4 Dyson R (1991) *Changing Labour Utilisation in NHS Trusts: the re-profiling paper.* University of Keele, Keele.
5 Health Services Management Unit (1996) *The Future Healthcare Workforce: the Steering Group Report.* HSMU, University of Manchester.
6 United Kingdom Central Council (1992) *Code of Professional Conduct.* UKCC, London.
7 United Kingdom Central Council (1992) *Scope of Professional Practice.* UKCC, London.
8 McWhinney IR (1997) *A Textbook of Family Medicine* (2nd ed). Oxford University Press, Oxford.
9 Department of Health (1994) *The Heathrow Debate.* DoH, London.
10 Welsh Office (1998) *NHS Wales: putting patients first.* The Stationery Office, London.
11 The Scottish Office (1997) *Designed to Care: renewing the National Health Service in Scotland.* The Stationery Office, Edinburgh.
12 Department of Health (1997) *The New NHS: modern, dependable.* The Stationery Office, London.

13 Department of Health (1998) *Our Healthier Nation: a contract for health.* The Stationery Office, London.

14 The Scottish Office (1998) *Working Together for a Healthier Scotland.* The Stationery Office, Edinburgh.

4

Integrated nursing teams and the PHCT: integral or alternative?

Glyn Elwyn and John Øvretveit

'Certain problems and behaviours will be encountered if the structure is wrong, regardless of who works in the structure. People come and go, but the problems will remain. Problems of structure are not overcome by calling a group a team.'[1]

Introduction: how have integrated nursing teams emerged?

Young described three actions to create 'integrated nursing':

'It involves devolving the nursing budget to the team level, removing hierarchical restrictions and implementing a training programme to enhance the change process and the self-management concept.'[2]

Young's paper, which discussed the concepts considered in this chapter, caused quite a stir when it appeared in a Royal College of Nursing publication, judging by the subsequent correspondence. Integrating nurses is clearly a controversial topic.

Forming a team composed of nurses (community, practice and health visitors) based on the practice list and location is a popular activity in the late 1990s. But integrated nursing teams (INTs), in primary care at least, have not suddenly appeared. They have developed within the primary healthcare team (PHCT), perhaps as a response to the structural problems faced by such teams. This chapter considers research into the organisation and working of PHCTs and discusses the implications for INTs and their future under the current reforms.

The history of interprofessional working in primary care helps us understand some of the future possibilities. The independent contractor status of the general practitioner was enshrined in the establishment of the NHS in 1948. In the early 1960s, a decision was made to 'attach' community staff (district nurses and, later, health visitors) to general practices to achieve a co-ordinated approach to issues such as care of the elderly and immunisation.[3] In the 1970s general practitioners, using ancillary staff allowances, began directly to employ practice nurses. The differing employment status of general practitioners, practice nurses and community nurses led to tensions between professionals assumed to form a team. Figure 4.1 demonstrates the additive nature of the process that has led to the current multidisciplinary complexity of the modern primary care organisation.

Year

1952   a

          a + 1/2b

          a + b

          a,n + b

          a,n + b,2n

1960   a,n + b,2n + (c)

          a,n + b,2n + (c)   + (d)

1970   a,n + b,2n + (c,m) + (d) (e)

          a,n + b,2n + (c,m) + (d,m) (e,m) + c

          a,n + b,m + (c,m) + (d,m) (e,m) + c + (f,m)

          a,n + b,m + (c,m) + (d,m) (e,m) + c,m + (f,m) + g,m

2002   a,n + b,m + (c,m) + (d,m) (e,m) + c,m + (f,m) + g,m

Key: Growth and development of PHCT where a = general practitioner, b = receptionist, c = nurse, d = nurse assistant, e = health visitor, f = other professions allied to medicine, g = practice manager, n = medical practices committee factor and m = multiple external management factor. Parentheses indicate attached staff.

Figure 4.1 The development of the PHCT.[4]

The term 'primary healthcare team' appeared in the 1970s[5] and it was thought initially that teamworking was likely to produce benefits.[6] However, the Cumberlege Report on community nursing stated that teams existed in name only and that the observed reality was a far cry from effective teamwork.[7] It identified poor interprofessional liaison and skill-mix problems among primary healthcare professionals. Particular difficulties arose from changes in the provision of community nursing services. Different disciplines were working in different communities and there was concern that 'neighbourhoods' were being built upon demographic and geographic grounds and not according to the needs of local populations.[8] Edwards suggested a solution – that all PHCTs should work within the same location and an action research project with all the PHCTs in Powys, Wales came to the same conclusion.[9,10]

The primary healthcare non-team

It was becoming clear, however, that the problems were about more than just location and geographical remit. Problems began to surface in the 1980s.[11,12] Bond et al. found low levels of collaboration between community staff and general practitioners;[13] McClure reported that interprofessional communication was often patient-specific rather than concerned with team objectives and processes;[11] and Wiles and Robinson and Cant and Killoran found a significant lack of integration between general practitioners, midwives and health visitors.[14,15] The awareness that collaboration in general practice-based primary care was more wish than substance was articulated most forcibly by Pearson in the early 1990s, when she used the term 'the primary healthcare non-team'.[16,17]

In 1990, a new contract was introduced for general practitioners. It contained payments linked to the achievement of targets in cervical screening, immunisation, surveillance of the over-75s and health promotion. Many of these tasks could potentially be delegated and there were hopes that the team would rise to these challenges, galvanised by the tasks set for them. The incentives were perceived, correctly, as financial for general practitioners and the work was consequently widely regarded as the responsibility of the practice and its employees. For this reason, among others, the ranks of the practice nurses have swelled significantly over the last decade – their direct employment by general practitioners facilitated the process of workload delegation and task substitution.

Working relationships also changed because of the fundholding scheme.[18] Many practices began to exert a degree of financial control over the provision of community services, influencing the working practice of district nurses and health visitors. Although contracts were drawn up which clearly stipulated teamworking aspirations within well-described service specifications, these hopes were often unaccomplished as community trust staff maintained previously established working methods.[19] Fundholding may have precipitated many local innovations, but it is questionable whether it assisted teamworking in a wider or sustainable way.[18]

It has been noted that primary healthcare organisations fail to set aside the time necessary to build teams. In addition, professional conflicts in terms of power, status and leadership assumptions lead to a lack of cohesiveness and team strategy.[10,20,21] When West and Poulton used well-validated measures of team functioning (clear objectives, participation in decision making, task orientation and support for innovation), to examine 68 practice teams, they found that PHCTs scored significantly lower than others such as social services teams and community mental health teams.[22,23] The very nature of teamworking in primary care has been questioned and calls have been made for a reassessment.[24]

Barriers to teamwork in primary care

What are the problems and barriers that impede teamwork in both primary healthcare and INTs? Many have been described – here we concentrate on the structural problems which we believe account for the more superficial symptoms reported. An action research study of all PHCTs in Powys in 1989 found that communication between professions concerning individual patients varied considerably.[10] The two main structural impediments to co-operation were the separate management and accountability structures of nursing and general medical practice, and the differing patient populations of both. Teams did not carry out some of the higher-level systems management, planning and needs assessment which were viewed as part of their task. This research distinguished between co-operation and integration in teamwork and noted a number of handicaps to co-operation between primary healthcare professionals.

The work reported barriers which included: no time allocated to team functioning; part-time working; large numbers of staff; different patient populations; different location bases and problems with base design; unclear roles and expertise of colleagues unknown; unclear case co-ordination arrangements; different professional policies; and differing management accountabilities. This work has been validated more recently by West and Field, West and Poulton and Pearson and Spencer who, having reviewed the literature, conclude that 'the context of primary healthcare is such that there are substantial barriers to co-operation and collaboration'.[21,23,25,26]

Scepticism about teams has not been confined to healthcare. Multinational companies have begun to question their benefit. Donnellon points to 'a mounting sense of disillusionment and even cynicism about teamwork' in industry, saying that the only tasks that necessitate teams of professional and managerial level employees are those which:

> 'Require the continuous integration of knowledge, experience, or perspective that cannot be found in one person but rather is distributed among several people.'[27]

There are other reasons for questioning the emphasis on teams in recent years, at least the need for large teams. Patients do not favour large teams in primary care. The personal element of primary care, the continuity of contact with a known community nurse, health visitor and general practitioner can disappear within an anonymous network of professionals. The problems of providing personal care in complex organisations are well described.[28-31] Consumers have different perspectives to practitioners. They prefer continuity, personal lists and small practices.[32] Large teams find it difficult to meet these preferences, especially when the structural problems have not been addressed. As a result, practices and professionals struggle with the team concept, with varying degrees of success.[33]

What solutions have been tried?

There are many teamworking projects and packages that have been developed for the primary care sector. Away-days and team development workshops, of differing intensity and quality, have been held in every region of the UK. It is a reflection of the *ad hoc* nature of this activity that there are no longitudinal studies that have objectively evaluated the effects of team development. West confirms that 'an important question remains unanswered: does teamwork in primary care actually make a difference to patient care, patient satisfaction or health outcomes? Research on this question is urgently needed'.[26]

There is, however, a general acknowledgement that the PHCT is too large and too ill-defined an organisation to be considered a cohesive entity. Different and sometimes piecemeal solutions are usually put forward by individual practices as part of local service developments, but are seldom subject to formal evaluation. No central policy or structural changes to tackle the lack of teamworking in primary care have emerged from the

NHS as yet, despite the importance of this issue to the primary health care organisations proposed in the NHS White Paper.

There are nevertheless examples of attempts to break the primary care network down into more manageable units. Many have been described in the popular press and examples are beginning to be appear in the academic literature.[34,35] The Four Elms Medical Centre in Cardiff proposed the term 'practice-based team' and in 1994 agreed a fundholding contract with the Premier Community Trust in Stoke-on-Trent to develop an integrated nursing team. The Wemsum Valley Medical Practice in Norwich introduced a nurse-led illness service and has developed small task-oriented teams within an overall practice-based contract with the health authority.[36] Similar work has been described at the Birchwood Medical Centre in Warrington.[37] The Lyme Regis Community Care Unit espouses the same philosophy and has a practice team directly employed by the community-based organisation.[38] As other chapters in this book illustrate, what started as tentative experiments by fundholding practices has led to a wave of similar ventures.

The development of a managed primary care organisation

From its origin as a service based around single practitioners, the NHS is moving towards a managed primary care service. This development is easily traced. In the 1970s, district nurses and health visitors were expected to liaise with nominated practices as part of their geographical remit – a process termed 'attachment' (*see* Figure 4.2).

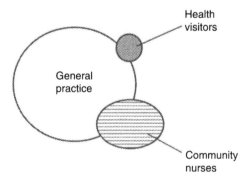

Figure 4.2 The 1970s attached staff model.[39]

As district nurses and health visitors were aligned with general practice they became a recognised part of the practice organisation – many were gradually provided with office space and other facilities – even though they were accountable to external management. But, as we have described, effective teamworking was impeded by organisational problems. The recognition of these structural barriers led to the concept of a representative core team being proposed and eventually debated nationally by the Royal College of General Practitioners.[39,40] Members from the three main domains – management, nursing and medicine – would, it was suggested, form an operational policy group, as illustrated by Figure 4.3.

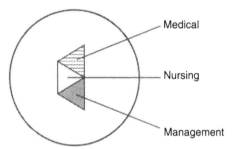

Figure 4.3 The 1990s core team model.[39]

The existence of this structured method of developing an operational policy (even if it only existed as a theoretical model) coupled with the added leverage that fundholding provided, led to a call for practice-based teams. What eventually evolved in many areas was a nursing team which has, in many regions, become known as an integrated nursing team (INT) – a team within an organisation, as illustrated by Figure 4.4.

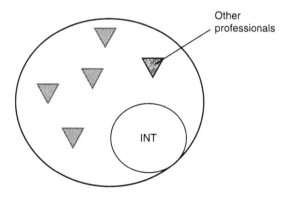

Figure 4.4 The INT in primary care.

Why the practice-based team should have become an INT deserves further enquiry. It is possible that size and cohesiveness may contribute to this phenomenon and there are sufficient numbers of nurses in primary care organisations to form groups of roughly five to nine individuals. It could be speculated that the development of INTs also reflects the greater commitment of nurses to the concept of teamwork – there is clearly room for further research here. As more practices engage in the process of developing an INT it is important to consider both the advantages and the potential problems which could occur.

The advantages and disadvantages of developing an INT

One clear advantage associated with the formation of an INT is that for the first time a team is defined, planned and managed in the primary care context. Benefits stem from the structured co-operation made transparent between disciplinary groups. As other chapters in this book indicate, an INT is a more formal arrangement than its part predecessor – the amorphous primary healthcare network.[1] The fundamental issue of team leadership is tackled. Team leader job descriptions exist and this pivotal role should be open to competition (in contrast to the assumed leadership in many previous arrangements). Membership of the team is defined and the work of the different nursing disciplines is discussed and agreed, with the overall aim of allowing role substitution where appropriate or sub-specialisation if indicated. The typical size of an INT is within the six to ten 'ideal' number for teamworking. Nursing has a long tradition of accepting formal leadership and the INT concept allows this type of function to reappear in a primary care arena. Regular meetings and detailed feedback against agreed task objectives are therefore far more likely to occur. In short, an INT is more likely to be a *managed* enterprise.

The potential disadvantages of an INT are those that occur when one profession retreats. As the roles and responsibilities of nurses are extended in primary care to involve triage, prescribing and chronic disease management, the distinction between doctors and nurses is becoming blurred although doctors retain their generalist role whilst nurses increasingly specialise. West suggested that between the medical and nursing professions there are:

'Deep historical professional divisions, exacerbated by gender differentiation, which characterise the primary healthcare context.'[26]

Will INTs exacerbate that divide? They certainly have the potential to segregate nurses from the general practice part of the organisation. If INTs see themselves as self-managing entities, practice management may find itself unable to engage with them and become unable to modify their service delivery. Even parts of the nursing community may begin to feel excluded. Community psychiatric nursing (and midwifery in many areas) is currently perceived to be an outreach service from secondary care. Are they to be included (or represented) in an INT?

How will doctors perceive the development of an INT? Have they been hoping all along to achieve a close involvement with the workload and roles of community nursing and health visiting only to see them close ranks, but now within the boundaries of general practice? How do they participate, if at all, in the management of the INT at practice or primary care organisation levels? How will nursing teams, without medical support, allow the nurse practitioner and nurse specialist roles to develop? Another concern is the impact the changes in primary care will have on INTs.[41] The identification of a separate community services budget was one of the most important factors that enabled the INT to be defined and managed. If community nursing budgets are abolished, will the *raison d'être* of the INT disappear? There is a danger that stronger nurse management in the new primary care groupings may weaken the practice-based links which INTs are achieving.

Primary care teams in the new NHS?

'Let a thousand flowers blossom' was one of the phrases used to describe the different arrangements in place for primary care organisations in the latter half of 1997. Fundholding, commissioning groups, multifunds, total purchasing consortia, health action zones and primary care agencies – are some of the labels used to describe the multitude of purchasing models in place. The 1997 White Paper, *The New NHS* indicates how the plethora of mechanisms created by the internal market are to be reshaped into a more collaborative NHS.[41] Locality commissioning is described as the proposed purchasing mechanism – a primary care group (drawing representatives from up to 50 GPs) will commission services for a population somewhere between 50 000–100 000.

It is unclear, however, how the shape of primary care provider function is to be developed. There is speculation that the umbrella organisation based on the locality commissioning unit (a type of primary care organisation or trust) will be responsible for controlling the number of outlets, for setting and monitoring standards, and for introducing a system of practice re-accreditation (perhaps using a health inspectorate service).[42] If this type of organisation does take shape, it would certainly be a clear move away from the corner-shop philosophy that has guided the planning of general practice-based primary care since its inception.

It is no surprise, therefore, that proposals are emerging which suggest that a salaried general practitioner service takes its place alongside others in an employed team, particularly in areas where recruitment is at its most difficult.[43] This gradual transition away from a small business model for general practice to a managed primary care service will, if it occurs, need to develop its structures carefully. As demand for healthcare continues to grow, role substitution must be planned and developed.[44] Teams will need to be managed as cohesive units delivering specific tasks and shaped around the one-stop concept where problems are presented, assessed and investigated in one location, in the shortest possible time frame.[45] Methods to ensure that patients receive adequate consulting time, and as much continuity of care as is practical will need to be established.[32,46–49] In addition, ways of providing quality assurance as an integral part of the work are required.[50] In industry this process has been termed 're-engineering' – an unhelpful term perhaps but the methods are as relevant to the delivery of healthcare as to any other service organisation.[34,51,52]

The reassessment of multidisciplinary teamwork in the UK is long overdue. Perhaps the time has come to recognise that patients do not benefit from large, fragmented, multiprofessional networks where professional tribalism impedes collaboration.[53] INTs might represent one of the steps along the path towards a managed primary healthcare service. Figure 4.5 outlines an organisation in which co-ordinated professional teams (CPTs) are formed and managed. At their intersection a small core group should be brought together to define an operational policy.

Within the wider organisation service delivery is undertaken either by individuals consulting with patients/clients or by task units, e.g. contraception service, cervical screening, child surveillance and immunisation service.

Building effective teams in the future

In this last section we consider how effective teamworking can be achieved as part of the new primary care organisation. INTs have demonstrated that it is possible to achieve a well-structured team in primary care. The

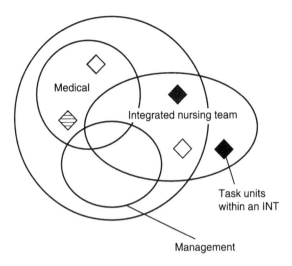

Medical

Integrated nursing team

Task units
within an INT

Management

A task may be multiprofessional and organised around a specific
service, e.g. child surveillance or immunisation. The different
shaded lozenges represent 'different' task units.

Figure 4.5 Integrated task teams in primary care.

changing face of the primary care sector in the UK at the end of the 1990s
may provide scope to build on this structured approach to teamworking.
The merger of authorities in 1995, unified budgets and new primary
healthcare groups now allow the possibility of developing unified management. History, however, should alert us against falling into the same
trap set for teams established from the 1970s onwards. The 1980s saw a
boom in community multidisciplinary teams but many were fraught with
problems. Research into teamwork in the mid-1980s found that the scepticism of some managers and clinicians was justified. Many early teams
were not planned and badly set up and managed and it is only over the last
few years that attention has been paid to the planning and maintenance
requirements of teams.[12]

Teams should be planned and managed: implications for INTs

Teams are best planned as part of a system of care based on an assessment of need. In the case of PHCTs, it has often been unclear who is responsible for planning and setting up the team. Responsibilities are often distributed across a number of managers, none of whom have clear co-ordinating responsibility. All too often the sequence of team formation is as follows:

- problems in teamwork
- attention to team organisation
- agreeing team operational policy and procedure
- clarification of services the team should offer
- adjustment of team services in relation to other services provided in the area
- assessment of needs of the population
- readjustment of team staffing mix in terms of grade and profession.

However, with the advent of emerging PCGs, the preferable and ideal approach to planning teams should be to start with an analysis of needs and end up with the details of team organisation as follows:

- assessment of the needs of the population
- plan the range of separate services to meet the most pressing needs
- describe the role and purpose of the team as a key part of the range of services, and where the team base will be
- describe the range of sub-services to be offered by the team
- decide which professionals and skills are required and the numbers of each
- agree the details of the extent of team organisation.

A key question for PCGs to ask is 'what type of team is required?' An INT is likely to be a network for co-ordinating separate professional services – a co-ordinated professional team – rather than a team where the services are a shared responsibility – a collective responsibility team.[24] There are many aspects to forming and developing close interprofessional working relationships in teams but insufficient attention is often paid to the two most simple and important considerations: a well-designed team base and an operational policy framework as outlined in Box 4.1.[1,24]

Box 4.1 Structural conditions for interprofessional co-operation in primary healthcare.[10]

At the practice level, attention needs to be paid to the following areas to create or develop multidisciplinary organisation – either an INT or a full PHCT. The more of the following essential conditions are present, the less dependent co-operation will be on the luck of the right mix of personalities.

1 Higher level manager/group responsible for improving co-operation or setting up a multidisciplinary team.

2 Align practitioner and patient populations, i.e. same geographical catchment and/or registration list.

3 Define practitioners' time available for teamwork, e.g. how much time working as part of the PHCT and how much working as part of other teams.

4 Common index of all patients currently served by and registered with each team member.

5 One office base for all members.

6 An agreed and defined team leader role with responsibilities, authority and accountability.

7 Explicit policy on:
   – procedure for allocation of work within the team once accepted
   – procedure for transfer of cases within the team (internal referral)
   – policy on how reviews will be done (team updates?)
   – closure policy and criteria.

8 Defined case co-ordinator role for cases involving more than one team member, and procedure for deciding and for changing case co-ordinator.

9 One patient – one case record file. Single record file with different records in it for easy access by team members.

10 Specification and agreement of other subjects which need to be covered in an operational policy which defines different members' roles, and includes other agreed procedures and policies binding all team members.

11 Regular review of policy – internally and with higher level management every six months or annually.

Conclusion

Integrated nursing teams are a phenomenon of the late 1990s.[54] The structural and organisational deficits inherent in the additive and unplanned way in which PHCTs have grown have been described and recognised. Many general practitioners were convinced that a more cohesive and co-ordinated team at practice level would deliver a better service. The market philosophy and the purchaser–provider split introduced into the NHS allowed them to experiment with practice-based teams and to specify contracts for INTs. Because of the largely unplanned nature of these developments their effect has not been objectively evaluated and there is little in the way of published evidence to suggest that either teamworking or the more recent development of INTs in primary care, lead to better outcomes for patients.

Multidisciplinary organisations can provide effective services where teams create operational policies and the issues of leadership, roles and responsibilities have been planned, agreed and are continuously managed.[55] INTs may be the tentative first step towards primary healthcare organisations which deliver managed care within a state funded system and it is unlikely to be the last we hear of teamwork in primary care.

References

1   Øvretveit J (1993) *Co-ordinating Community Care.* Open University Press, Milton Keynes.
2   Young L (1997) Improved primary care through integrated nursing. *Primary Health Care.* 7:8–10.
3   Pinsent RJ, Pike LA, Morgan RH *et al.* (1961) The health visitor in general practice. *BMJ.* 1:123–7.
4   Stott NCH (1993) When something is good, more of the same is not always better. *Brit J Gen Prac.* 43:254–7.
5   British Medical Association (1974) *Primary Healthcare Teams.* BMA, London.
6   Harding W and Frost W (1981) *The Primary Healthcare Team: report of the Standing Medical Advisory Committee and Standing Nursing and Midwifery Advisory Committee.* DHSS, London.
7   Cumberlege J (1986) *Neighbourhood Nursing: a focus for care.* DHSS, London.

8   Dalley G (1990) The impact of new community management structures: an overview. In: J Hughes (ed) *Enhancing The Quality of Community Nursing*. King's Fund, London.

9   Edwards D (1987) *Nursing in The Community: a team approach for Wales. Report of the review of community nursing*. Welsh Office, Cardiff.

10 Øvretveit J (1990) *Improving Primary Healthcare Team Organisation*. Research Report, BIOSS. Brunel University, Uxbridge.

11 McClure LM (1984) Teamwork: myth or reality. Community nurses' experience with general practice attachment. *J Epidemiol and Comm Health*. **31**:68–74.

12 Øvretveit J (1986) *Organising Multidisciplinary Community Teams*. HCS Working Paper, BIOSS. Brunel University, Uxbridge.

13 Bond J, Cartilidge AM, Gregson BA *et al*. (1985) *A Study of Inter-professional Collaboration in Primary Care. Report No 27*. University of Newcastle upon Tyne, Health Care Research Unit, Newcastle upon Tyne.

14 Wiles R and Robinson J (1994) Teamwork in primary care: the views and experience of nurses, midwives and health visitors. *J Advanced Nursing*. **20**:324–30.

15 Cant S and Killoran A (1993) Team tactics: a study of nurse collaboration in general practice. *Health Education J*. **52**:203–8.

16 Pearson P and van Zwanenberg T (1991) *Who is the Primary Healthcare Team? What should they be doing?* University of Newcastle upon Tyne, Department of Primary Care, Newcastle upon Tyne.

17 Pearson P (1994) The primary healthcare non-team? *BMJ*. **309**:1387–8.

18 Audit Commission (1996) *Fundholding: the main report*. Audit Commission, London.

19 Jones Elwyn G and Marsh HM (1995) Practice-based Teamworking. *Four Elms Medical Centre*. Service Specification for the Bro Taf Health Authority, Cardiff.

20 Poulton BC and West MA (1993) Effective multidiscipinary teamwork in primary health care. *J Advanced Nursing*. **18**:918–25.

21 West M and Field R (1994) Teamwork in primary care 1. Perspectives from organisational psychology. *J Interprof Care*. **9**:117–22.

22 Anderson NR and West M (1994) *The Team Climate Inventory: manual and users' guide*. ASE Press, Windsor.

23 West M and Poulton BC (1997) A failure of function: teamwork in primary healthcare. *J Interprof Care*. **11**:205–16.

24 Øvretveit J, Mathias P and Thompson T (1997) *Interprofessional Working in Health and Social Care*. Macmillan, Basingstoke.

25 Pearson P and Spencer J (eds) (1997) *Promoting Teamwork in Primary Care: a research-based approach*. Arnold, London.

26 West M and Slater J (1995) *The Effectiveness of Teamworking in Primary Healthcare*. Health Education Authority, London.
27 Donellon A (1996) *Team Talk*. Harvard Business School Press, Boston.
28 Stott NCH (1995) Personal care and teamwork: implications for the general practice-based primary healthcare team. *J Interprof Care*. **9**: 95–101.
29 Williamson V (1995) Personal care and teamwork in primary care: the patient perspective. *J Interprof Care*. **9**:101–7.
30 Sawyer B (1995) Personal care and teamworking. *J Interprof Care*. **9**: 107–13.
31 Freeman G (1995) Towards the millennium: personal care and the primary healthcare team. *J Interprof Care*. **9**:113–17.
32 Baker R (1995) What type of general practice do patients prefer? Exploration of practice characteristics influencing patient satisfaction. *Brit J Gen Prac*. **45**:654–9.
33 Robinson J and Wiles R (1993) Building teamwork: the value of the multidisciplinary meeting. *Primary Care Management*. **3**:9–11.
34 Jones Elwyn G, Rapport FL and Kinnersley P (1997) Re-engineering the primary health care team. *J Interprof Care*. **12**:189–98.
35 Meads G (ed) (1996) *Future Options for General Practice*. Radcliffe Medical Press, Oxford.
36 Lister A (1996) How I inspired the general practice revolution. *Pulse*. **Nov**:2–3.
37 Editorial (1996) Triage helps general practitioner to focus care. *Medeconomics*. **Dec**:53.
38 Robinson B (1996) Primary managed care: the Lyme alternative. In: G Meads (ed) *Future Options for General Practice*. Radcliffe Medical Press, Oxford.
39 Thomas D (1994) *Developing Fully Integrated Primary Healthcare Teams: discussion paper for the Primary Care Development Group*. Welsh Chief Executives Group, Cardiff.
40 Royal College of General Practitioners Working Party (1996) *The Nature of General Practice*. RCGP, London.
41 Secretary of State for Health (1997) *The New NHS: modern, dependable*. The Stationery Office, London.
42 Oldham J (1997) An inspectorate for the health service? *BMJ*. **315**: 896–7.
43 Tudor Hart J (1997) *Going for Gold: a new approach to primary medical care in the South Wales Valleys*. A Socialist Health Association Discussion Paper. UNISON, Swansea.
44 Warner MM (1991) *Health Strategy for the 1990s: five areas for substitution*. *Healthcare UK*. King's Fund, London.

45 Consumers' Association (1993) *Getting To See Your General Practitioner*. Consumers' Association, London.

46 Williams SJ and Calnan M (1991) Key determinants of consumer satisfaction. *Family Practice*. **8**:237–42.

47 Wilson A (1991) Consultation length in general practice: a review. *Brit J Gen Prac*. **41**:119–22.

48 Howie JGR, Porter AMD, Heaney DJ and Hopton JL (1991) Long to short consultation ratio: a proxy measure of quality of care for general practice. *Brit J Gen Prac*. **41**:48–54.

49 Baker R (1996) Characteristics of practices: general practitioners and patients related to levels of patients' satisfaction with consultations. *Brit J Gen Prac*. **46**:601–5.

50 Øvretveit J (1991) *Primary Care Quality Through Teamwork*. Research Report, BIOSS. Brunel University, Uxbridge.

51 Øvretveit J (1994) A framework for cost-effective team quality. *J Interprof Care*. **8**:329–33.

52 Merry P (1996) Back to the drawing board. *Medical Interface*. **August**: 11–14.

53 Hunter DJ (1996) The changing roles of health personnel in health and healthcare management. *Soc Sci Med*. **43**:799–808.

54 Jones Elwyn G (1997) *Integrated Nursing Teams in Primary Care*. Conference proceedings. Clinical Effectiveness Support Unit, Cardiff.

55 Øvretveit J (1997) Planning and managing teams. *Health and Social Care*. **5**(4):269–83.

5

Professional training issues for integrated nursing teams

June Smail

Introduction: the scope of community healthcare nursing, education and practice

There are a number of recent educational developments in community nursing that will change practice. The first is the trend towards greater autonomy, accountability and removal of restrictions to practice which has been firmly outlined in the United Kingdom Central Council for Nursing, Midwifery and Health Visiting (UKCC) document, *Scope of Professional Practice*.[1] The second development, nurse prescribing, will follow this trend towards greater efficiency and professional accountability, and the third and possibly greatest influence will be the UKCC's *Standards for Education and Practice Following Registration*.[2,3]

The UKCC affirms that nurses, midwives and health visitors practise in an environment which is subject to constant change in relation to the organisation of services, boundaries and delivery of care and technological advances in treatment and care. Influences on education have also developed around the growing concerns about educational standards and fitness to practise, recruitment and retention of students and skill-mix in primary care.

The future community healthcare nurse (CHCN)

The UKCC has a primary legislative function to establish and improve standards of education, training and professional conduct for all those on its register – approximately 640 000 registrants. The UKCC began its work on education standards in 1986 with a review of pre-registration nursing and midwifery education, which became known as *Project 2000*.[4]

Attention then focused on educational standards for post-registration education and practice (PREP) and in 1994 the UKCC described a new and unified discipline of community healthcare nursing.[5] This discipline reflects the core skills required for all community nurses as well as the additional specialist skills required for discrete areas of practice.

From October 1998, nurses who wish to work in the community as a CHCN will undertake a specialist programme of education at degree level, structured around a common core. Two-thirds of the programme will be common to all community nurses, thereby encouraging a more generalist approach to their roles and responsibilities. One-third of the programme will then be taught in the specialist community areas of:

- general practice nursing

- home nursing (district nursing)

- public health nursing (health visiting)

- community mental health nursing

- community mental handicap (learning disabilities)

- school nursing

- community paediatric nursing

- occupational health nursing.

These changes in education and practice will bring together all nurses working in the community, to demonstrate that there is unity in the diversity of practice. In future, all community nurses should have a clearer understanding of 'generalist' roles and those pertaining to discrete areas of practice. The challenge to educators and practitioners alike calls for a flexible approach which removes unnecessary barriers in practice and overlaps in educational preparation, thus promoting improved understanding and communication. Box 5.1 highlights the four principles adopted for the community focus within PREP.

Although these new programmes of community education will be mandatory from October 1998 to allow practice at specialist level, those district and practice nurses, health visitors, school nurses and other community disciplines currently in practice will not be required to undertake further qualifications in order to continue practising. Each nurse will have

---

Box 5.1   Principles adopted for community nursing within PREP.

1 The need to build upon the contributions of current community nursing skills whilst providing a vision for the future of community nursing.

2 The provision of a logical and cost-effective approach to education.

3 Removal of unnecessary barriers to practise and overlaps in preparation, to enable nursing to continue to make an effective contribution to the care and health of communities.

4 Recognition of the need to prepare practitioners for work in the community following the completion of *Project 2000* courses.

---

to make a decision based on their career aspirations and the demands of their current role, as to whether to pursue a specialist qualification in community nursing. However, there is a requirement for all nurses to undertake continuing education as outlined in *PREP and You*.[6]

Developing a teamworking ethos in community nursing

This new framework for community education should remove a number of barriers to teamwork in primary care.[7-10] Many of the training issues within teams – understanding roles, relationships and responsibilities, profiling and planning to meet community health needs, clinical leadership and management skills – will all be addressed in the common core programme.

The ability to work in teams is a skill that can be learnt, provided individuals are prepared to make the effort. The benefits should become apparent as better care for patients, greater job satisfaction for staff, higher team morale and a greater sense of achievement. Effective teamworking requires that the team members feel comfortable with the idea of working more closely and harmoniously together. It is essential that all team members value each other for the important contributions that they make. In this way, the working relationships can be positive and equitable, rather than allowing professional rivalries to take precedence.

Research studies confirm that nurses have a greater commitment to the concept of teamwork than doctors.[11,12] Belbin's team role theory frequently identifies nurses as team workers.[13] Some community nurses, with a great deal of energy and often against the odds, are achieving positive change.[14] Generally, community nurses have accepted that integrated nursing is a good way forward and we have the experience of a number of teams to draw upon. Where integrated nursing teams (INTs) have worked well the benefits have been:

- greater flexibility between community nurses

- increased nurse autonomy and confidence

- more responsive client-centred services

- a more supportive environment where communication and relationships are continually improved.[14]

How can facilitation help develop and train primary care teams?

The first step to successful team development is to identify a team facilitator.[15] Although a framework for INTs/primary care teams should be based on the principle that direction and coherence should come from within the team, external facilitation can enable progress without being perceived as directive.

The principles underlying the model developed in Southampton were:[15]

- that the key expertise of facilitators is their ability to enable individuals to work together effectively and to manage change well

- that the facilitator should first consult with those to who she/he would be of service

- that in order to be most effective, the facilitator should remain neutral and enable the team to make their own decisions

- that the lessons learned from facilitation in industrial settings could successfully be applied to primary care.

Responses from 166 practice team members to a questionnaire on the importance of aspects of the facilitator role in teambuilding demonstrated that maintaining enthusiasm, helping teams plan the future, helping members expand their roles and agree responsibilities, being an educational resource and resolving differences and developing clinical policies, protocols and audit were all rated as very important.[15] This study also examined the concept of 'readiness to change'. Individuals rated their own readiness to change significantly higher than that of their practice. Overall, 59% of responders rated themselves as very ready to change. In contrast, the same responders rated 30% of their practices as ready to change.

There is evidence from descriptive service-based projects that effective change management requires careful facilitation and that teambuilding workshops can be effective in improving team processes.[16–19]

Identifying training needs for INTs

Although INT models may vary, there is agreement that the following criteria are important features of successful initiatives:

- the practice needs to develop a population needs analysis, set priorities for practice and develop shared objectives around these priorities

- the skill-mix of the team should reflect practice objectives

- there should be clear lines of management accountability within the team

- a clearly defined budget needs to be devolved to practice level

- objectives should be monitored to inform practice development

- the whole process requires careful facilitation and evaluation.

Training and facilitation will initially need to cover population health needs assessment and understand the roles and responsibilities of team members.[20] Other key areas which have been identified as training issues are:[21,22]

- personal, professional and clinical practice development

- factors in team development, change and risk management

- team leadership and self-management skills

- quality, audit and clinical effectiveness

- multidisciplinary learning in teams

- nurse prescribing

- NHS policy and organisational changes.

It must be recognised that practice and nursing teams are at various stages of development and a skilled facilitator will work to identify training needs, both of the team as a whole and of individuals. For this process to be successful, teams require protected time away from the practice. It is important that the team is encouraged to plan its own agenda and this should be seen as a part of the learning process. The facilitator has a key role in achieving knowledge transfer and in the development of co-operation between the team members. For facilitation to be most successful it should be independent from the organisations it is trying to help.[8] Box 5.2 sets out an overall aim and learning outcomes planned by a motivated team for an away day.

Box 5.2   Motivated team outcomes.

Overall aim: To determine shared goals and priorities towards self-management.

Learning outcomes: By the end of the day the team will have:

■ determined the roles and responsibilities of its members

■ identified the training needs required to take on those roles and responsibilities

■ set goals and priorities for the practice, team and individuals

■ identified what stage it has reached towards self-management

■ chosen the model of self-management it wishes to adopt

■ identified the team leader.

A dysfunctional team is frequently characterised by a blaming culture and members working in isolation. Such a team requires a basic understanding of teamworking before it can aspire to the outcomes described in Box 5.2. A more appropriate introductory session is described in Box 5.3.

Skill-mix in primary care

The concept of skill-mix is widely recognised by the NHS workforce.[23] However, it is a term without precise definition, used variously to refer to the mix of disciplinary groups involved in the delivery of a service, the mix of skills within a given disciplinary group and the mix of skills possessed by an individual.

Box 5.3 Introductory group working.

Overall aim: To explore the benefits of and barriers to good teamworking.

Learning outcomes: By the end of the session the team will have:

■ compared their views to the benefits and barriers to teamworking

■ discovered whether the benefits outweigh the snags

■ decided whether there are any barriers which can be addressed

■ developed a clearer idea of what teamwork means to them

■ agreed the ground rules for subsequent sessions.

At a time of rapid changes in primary care provision, the implementation of appropriate skill-mix in PHCTs becomes even more elusive. In order to address skill-mix issues it is essential to ascertain what team members actually do, how this may be changed, and assess the acceptability of spreading workload more effectively among other members of the team. Understanding roles and responsibilities is the first step in this process. There are two conceptually different ways in which changes in skill-mix are perceived to alter primary healthcare provision – delegation/substitution and diversification.[24]

Delegation/substitution

Tasks formerly performed by one type or grade of professional are transferred to a different type or grade of professional. Examples include delegation from GPs to senior nurses, and from senior nurses to junior nurses or nurse assistants. The intention is to reduce costs and improve service efficiency (*see* Chapter 2 for in-depth discussion on substitution).

Diversification

The range of services provided within primary care is enhanced through new types of professionals or through the acquisition of new skills of existing professionals. The intention is to fill previously unmet health needs and/or relocate services previously provided within hospitals or other settings.

In practice, skill-mix may involve both aspects. Ideally, skill-mix changes should be governed by evidence of how skills may be best distributed among health professionals, to improve the cost effectiveness of the health service. However, there is a dearth of research in this area and many innovations in skill-mix have not yet been adequately evaluated.

One study examined the constraints upon and opportunities for spreading the GP workload more effectively among members of the PHCT.[25] Attitudes to delegation and proxy outcomes were also measured. A study in Cardiff reported the acceptability of a practice nurse who saw patients with acute minor illnesses presenting in one general practice.[26] Although skill-mix developments in nursing have been the subject of preliminary studies, there is a need for much more research in this area.[27,28]

Insufficient attention has also been given to the impact of ongoing and proposed NHS reforms on the professional values, skill-mix and capacity for change within PHCTs.

Multidisciplinary/interprofessional education

The 1996 White Paper, *Primary Care: delivering the future*, points out that achieving quality in primary care will require interprofessional working.[29] It urges that a greater proportion of all education and training should be multidisciplinary and that specific training events to promote teamworking be provided in order to achieve this. Education, it notes, plays a significant role in forming attitudes. The failure to collaborate results from different training structures, ideologies and educational approaches. Evaluations of shared learning initiatives have looked at attitudinal change and have shown that after participation in even quite short programmes, professionals develop a greater understanding and valuing of other professionals.[30-32] Trust and respect for each other is also increased.

Funnell's review summarises the perceived benefits of multidisciplinary education as:[33]

- enhancing understanding of the roles and perceptions of other professions

- promoting teamwork and co-operation between professionals

- contributing to the learner's knowledge

- enhancing the acquisition and development of practical skills.

There are, therefore, strong arguments in favour of multidisciplinary education.[34] It is generally held that learning together will improve team-working and mutual understanding. Benefits, particularly at post-registration level, have been demonstrated. More emphasis on specific skills and knowledge needed to manage the complexities of the community setting will increase understanding among all groups, as well as promote self-esteem and mutual interdependence.[35]

> 'Doctors and nurses can both benefit if their relationship becomes more mutually interdependent. Subservient and dominant roles are both psychologically restricting. When a subordinate becomes liberated, there is potential for the dominant role to become liberated too'.[35]

Conclusion

Nurse educationalists have it within their power to change the culture of nursing in primary care.[36] Multidisciplinary education and the training for the new and unified discipline of community healthcare nursing should go some way to changing the attitudinal and organisational barriers which impede teamworking. But collaborative learning will need to start early in professional life. To prevent negative stereotypes developing about other professions, it is preferable to introduce shared learning at the start of education. Although the question of which educational approach best facilitates collaboration needs further research, it should at least be taking shape in our organisations.

The Centre for Advanced Interprofessional Education (CAIPE) has summarised a number of key characteristics of effective interprofessional education which include:[37]

- enhanced practice within professions

- improved quality of care

- increased professional satisfaction.

The UKCC has recently commissioned work into multiprofessional education and the Welsh Office also set up a taskforce for continuing education and practice in nursing, midwifery and health visiting in 1997.[38,39] The task force has recommended that an agenda for education needs to be drawn up which reviews educational arrangements to ensure a primary care and interprofessional focus, and places more emphasis on specific skills and knowledge needed to manage the complexities of the community setting.

The latest Government reforms place a greater emphasis than ever before on the whole culture and development of effective teamworking – but teams do not just happen.[40] Appreciation of each other's values is a basic motivating factor in team behaviour and an essential ingredient in morale.[8] Successful teams are achieved through skilled facilitation and a high level of participation and commitment by all members.

References

1   UKCC (1992) *Scope of Professional Practice*. UKCC, London.
2   Luker K (1996) *Evaluation of Nurse Prescribing*. University of Liverpool, Liverpool.
3   UKCC (1994) *Standards for Education and Practice Following Registration*. UKCC, London.
4   UKCC (1986) *Project 2000 – a new preparation for practice*. UKCC, London.
5   UKCC (1994) *Post-registration Education and Practice* (PREP). UKCC, London.
6   UKCC (1997) *PREP and You*. UKCC, London.
7   West M (1994) *Effective Teamwork, Personal and Professional Development*. BPS Books, Leicester.
8   Pritchard P and Pritchard J (1994) *Teamwork for Primary and Shared Care*. Oxford University Press, Oxford.
9   Wiles R and Robinson J (1994) Teamwork in primary care: the views and experiences of nurses, midwives and health visitors. *J Advanced Nursing*. **20**:324–30.
10 Cook R (1996) Paths to effective teamwork in primary care settings. *Nursing Times*. **92**:44–5.
11 Reid T and David A (1994) Primary care nursing: community nursing practice management and teamwork. *Nursing Times*. **90**:42–5.
12 Heath I (1994) Skill mix in primary care: should be used to match services to needs rather than to cut costs. *BMJ*. **308**:993–4.
13 Belbin R (1993) *Team Roles at Work: a strategy for human resource management*. Butterworth Heinemann, Oxford.
14 Young L (1997) Improved primary care through integrated nursing. *Primary Health Care*. **7**:8–10.
15 Speigal N (1994) How can facilitators help primary care teams? A distinct consultation. *J Interprof Care*. **8**:299–309.

16 Mayon-White B (1993) *Problem Solving in Small Groups: team members as agents of change*. Paul Chapman Publishing and Open University, London.

17 White D, Leach K and Christensen L (1996) Self-fulfilling prophecies. *Health Service Journal*. **2**:31.

18 Wiltshire Health Authority (1996) *Primary Care Nursing: a framework for action*. Wiltshire Health Authority, Swindon.

19 Poulton B (1997) *Evaluation of Practice-based Teams Project*. RCN, London.

20 Royal College of Nursing (1993) *The GP Practice Population Profile*. RCN, London.

21 Poulton B (1996) *Effective Multidisciplinary Teamwork in Primary Health Care*. RCN Paper 10. RCN, London.

22 Smail J (1996) *An Exploration of an Integrated Team Approach in Primary Health Care*. BA (Hons) Dissertation, University of Wales. Unpublished.

23 Jenkins-Clarke S, Carr-Hill R, Dixon P *et al*. (1997) *Skill-mix in Primary Care: a study of the interface between the GP and other members of the primary health care team*. University of York, York.

24 Sergison B, Sibbald B and Rose S (1997) *Skill-mix in Primary Care: a bibliography*. National Primary Care Research and Development Centre, Manchester.

25 Jenkins-Clarke S (1996) *Dilemmas of Delegation and Diversification*. Centre for Health Economics, University of York, York.

26 Rees M and Kinnersley P (1996) Nurse-led management of minor illnesses in a GP surgery. *Nursing Times*. **92**:32–3.

27 McKenna H (1995) Nursing skill-mix substitutions and quality of care. *J Advanced Nursing*. **21**:452–9.

28 Rashid A, Watts A, Lenehan C *et al*. (1996) Skill-mix in primary care: sharing workload and understanding professional roles. *Brit J Gen Prac*. **46**:639–40.

29 Department of Health (1996) *Primary Care: delivering the future*. DoH, London.

30 Carpenter J (1995) *Interprofessional Education for Medical and Nursing Students*. Blackwell Scientific, Oxford.

31 Carpenter J and Hewstone M (1996) Shared learning for doctors and social workers. *Brit J of Social Work*. **26**:239–57.

32 Gill J and Ling J (1994) Interprofessional shared learning: a curriculum for collaboration. In: K Soothill, L Mackay and C Webb (eds) *Interprofessional Relations in Healthcare*. Edward Arnold, London.

33 Funnell P (1994) Exploring the value of interprofessional shared learning. In: K Soothill, L Mackay and C Webb (eds) *Interprofessional Relations in Healthcare*. Edward Arnold, London.

34 Tope R (1996) *Integrated Interdisciplinary Learning Between the Health and Social Care Professions*. Avebury, Hampshire.

35 Stein L, Watt S and Howell T (1990) The doctor–nurse game revisited. *NEJM*. **322**:546–9.

36 Ford P and Walsh M (1995) *New Rituals for Old: nursing through the looking glass*. Butterworth-Heinemann, London.

37 Centre for Advanced Interprofessional Education (1997) *Effective Interprofessional Education*. CAIPE, London.

38 UKCC (1997) *Multiprofessional Education*. JEC/97/21. UKCC, London.

39 The Welsh Office (1997) *Task Force for Continuing Education and Practice: on the millennium threshold*. Welsh Office, Cardiff.

40 Department of Health (1997) *The New NHS: modern, dependable*. The Stationery Office, London.

6
Nursing roles in integrated teams

Kate Harris

Nurses working in primary care have accepted well defined roles, related to their professional background and education, i.e. health visiting, district nursing, midwifery and practice nursing. Although these roles have evolved over time as a response to many demands, the degree of role change is affected by a complex set of variables which include the expectations of management, general practitioners and patients. The composition of practice populations and the purchasing power of general practitioners has had an effect on nursing roles at the practice level. At a macro-level the availability of information to patients on what they can expect from health-care, the changing political climate, an ageing population and scarce resources, has also had an effect on the roles of nurses.

The Roy Report was a significant contribution to the policy debate about community nursing in the early 1990s.[1] The report suggested five different models of delivery for primary care nursing and stimulated a variety of project-based responses. One project in Wiltshire concentrated on the 'model' where general practitioners employ all the nursing staff providing care for their patients.[2] This was not an easy process. General practitioners were not confident that they knew exactly what community nurses did once a referral had been made. In order to consider employing this group of staff they needed more management information about exact role and caseloads.

Recognising that limitations were necessary, the project's aim was to identify the roles and activities of different nursing disciplines involved in general practice. The proposed outcomes were:

- the identification of nursing priorities
- the identification of skills to meet these priorities
- the identification of gaps and overlaps in nursing service provision

- a set of recommendations for addressing the gaps and overlaps in nursing provision including changes in the structure of the management organisation.

The results of this work demonstrated that facilitated nursing teams were indeed able to achieve the stated objectives and allow successful change to occur.[2] The results of this project have influenced ongoing work with primary care nursing teams in Wiltshire. It is now agreed:

- that nursing teams need facilitation to ensure constructive development
- that teamwork is the key to the delivery of an effective service
- nursing teams should identify nursing priorities, necessary skills, gaps and overlaps
- that a single line of management improves team functioning
- that organisational needs can be resolved within such teams.

An evolving integrated nursing team (INT) should be careful not to ignore patient demand and the practice population. It is essential that they carry out a baseline health needs assessment of the practice population, and a review of the services they currently provide. Some members of the team may not have had the opportunity to co-ordinate their knowledge when working together to identify health needs.

The following questions represent a health needs assessment criteria checklist.

1 Is the topic of relevance and importance?

2 Is the health need achievable within available resources?

3 Is there an easily identifiable group of patients?

4 Are there recognisable benefits to the community?

5 Are there effective interventions the team can use?

6 How much extra energy is needed by the team to achieve success?

7 How important is it to the whole community?

Using these criteria enables the nursing team to identify priorities and match these to the team skills, or make sure that new skills are developed. Health needs should also be linked to the strategic direction of the practice but also take account of local and national policies. Wiltshire Health Authority provides an example based on the following key themes:

- providing care at home or as near home as possible
- promoting integrated patient-centred care
- purchasing on a locality basis.

The project provided a developmental framework that is available for all future nursing initiatives.[2] This framework ensures a co-ordinated, effective and flexible use of the nursing resource to the practice population. The principles underpinning this approach can encompass a wider team membership than nurses, being dynamic enough to be used by health and social care teams. This ensures a flexible response to the diversity of general practice.

Nursing roles

Using a framework that enables a nursing team to identify the current roles of its team members is essential if they are to integrate successfully. The following steps are suggested:

- clarify roles and responsibilities
- develop a workload audit tool
- prioritise the workload
- develop skill-mix
- formulate an action plan
- inform the practice planning process.

Identifying nursing processes results in these activities being easily divided into two categories: shared skills and specific skills. Shared skills identified can be listed under the following headings:

- communication skills and good interpersonal relationships
- infection control
- health promotion
- wound management.

This list may vary from team to team. The shared skills are present in varying degrees directly related to the level of knowledge and expertise of the individual team members. Specific skills that may be identified overlap with some shared skills due to specialist knowledge in general areas. Specific skills can be listed as:

- an ability to assess the health needs of the practice population and provide a profile of that population

- wound management knowledge including evidence-based care of leg ulcers

- incontinence management, including assessment, diagnosis and treatment

- chronic disease management, e.g. asthma or epilepsy care

- child developmental surveillance

- infant feeding

- child protection

- counselling (recognised by the British Association of Counselling)

- minor operations (assisting)

- pain control knowledge for the care of palliative and chronic conditions

- cardiovascular disease risk assessment

- alternative therapies, such as acupuncture, reflexology and aromatherapy.

A study in the Netherlands on community nursing roles in teams consisting of members functioning at different levels demonstrated varying levels of skills.[3] They categorised nurses as being at first and second levels. In the UK, the first level would equate to registered general nurse or health visitor and the second level to a nursing auxillary. Their findings showed that 'assessment' and 'diagnosis' were attributes of first level nurses whilst second level nurses were involved with nursing tasks and processes. When comparing 'specialist' against 'generalist' skills, they demonstrated that generalist work by first level nurses was decreasing. Nurses had to choose either 'curative' adult care or 'preventative' mother and childcare. This compares, respectively, with district nurse and health visitor roles. They also concluded that the first and second level nurses could develop specialist skills in response to patient needs, if appropriate education and training was provided. They recommended a skill-mix of staff who would be able to respond to the nursing needs of the practice population. Within their recommendations was the expectation that nursing teams would use their expertise to meet identified health needs within a co-ordinated approach. This study provides a parallel to other work on INTs. It also reinforces the need to identify shared skills, specific skills and the levels at which they are applied in patient care and there are implications for professional development within the UKCC *Scope of Professional Practice* document.[4]

Another document that contributes to the issues surrounding the development of nursing roles in primary care is *The Development of Nursing and Health Visiting Roles in Clinical Practice* produced by the North Thames Region.[5] This investigative document came about as a response to the Government's emphasis on service delivery within the primary care sector and the impact this was having on nursing practice. The report linked this trend to the future education needs and professional support of primary care nurses. The document identified emerging role categories (*see* Box 6.1) and then linked them to competencies (*see* Box 6.2).

Box 6.1   Emerging role categories.

■ Doctor's assistant/replacement.

■ Clinical specialists.

■ Minor surgery and treatment (both carrying out and assisting).

■ Primary care practitioners – patients self-refer in the same way as they consult their general practitioner. The nurse prescribes within agreed protocols.

Box 6.2   Common competencies identified.

■ Physical assessment, screening and diagnosis.*

■ Pharmacology and drug interactions.*

■ Emotional support and counselling.

■ Referral and discharge.

■ Case management.

■ Applying research and audit to practice.

* Identified as new roles.

Physical assessment, screening and diagnosis and an understanding of pharmacology and drug interactions had not been identified as nursing competencies until now. But they have been determined by nurses responding to patient and service demands and the UKCC's *Scope of Professional Practice*.[4] The emergence of these roles and associated competencies lead to many unresolved questions about the future of nursing practice. A few of the issues that emerge when expanded roles are fostered are listed below.

Nursing assessment

What is the degree of physical assessment, screening and diagnosis at each level of nursing? Does the first level nurse take responsibility for this and then direct the nursing tasks and processes of the second level nurse?

Counselling skills

Should everyone in the team be using counselling or listening skills? Can team members articulate the difference between counselling and listening skills?

Nursing audit

Most people feel they are applying standards and carrying out audit. Can they demonstrate this by production of criteria, standards and audit results? Are these research based? Are standards regularly reviewed and audit recommendations implemented?

Administration or prescribing

Most team members administer medication or injections. Is this the same as being competent in pharmacology and drug interactions? What are the training requirements of a 'prescribing' role in nursing?

Supervision and professional development

What education and clinical supervision do nursing team members need to perform effectively?

Referral and case management

Whose responsibility are these areas? Are they related to current skills and targeted populations, i.e. health visitors and under fives, district nurses and the elderly, community psychiatric nurses adults and elderly care, midwives, antenatal and postnatal care, practice nurses, the over 75s?

Shared records and guidelines

This should always be explored to assist communication between professionals, carers and patients.

When new roles are being developed within INTs it is important to retain flexibility in the face of expressed demand. Team members will be more confident about breaking down traditional role boundaries if they have had the opportunity to identify current roles in relation to their existing competencies and the specific new skills required. Any gaps or overlaps revealed will need sensitive expansion and curtailment of services. The identification of training needs and a carefully facilitated consensus between team members will be needed to allow these changes to be successfully implemented.

Nursing teams working towards an integrated approach have demonstrated that overlaps and duplication can be minimised by:

- improved communication

- development of joint protocols

- computerisation and sharing of records

- multidisciplinary training

- development of peer group support and clinical supervision

- identification of lead nurses for priority health needs, i.e. family planning, child health surveillance, leg ulcer management and infection control.

Team leadership: necessary or not?

Even the most rudimentary team development will result in the identification of health needs and the importance of role clarity – but how can this initial teamworking be maintained and sustained? West and Pillinger's evaluation gives us some clues about team maintenance, one of which is the development of a leadership role.[6]

Do teams require leadership? It has been clearly demonstrated that the most effective teams have recognised leaders. A team can be described as 'a group in which the individuals share a common aim and in which the job and skills of each member fit in with those of the others'. Teams without leadership are made up of individuals going about their work without communicating with their colleagues. This approach can lead to inappropriate care for patients, e.g.

- a family receiving several home visits in one week from several different members of the team

- a request for help being ignored due to the lack of communication and an attitude of 'this is not my job'.

Lack of leadership may lead to inadequate measures of outcomes. Nurse managers, external to the group, may be able to pick up some leadership tasks but this can cause confusion between team members about the nature of their own decision-making processes. Clear leadership enables teams to fulfil the criteria for effectiveness suggested by West and Pillinger:[6]

- clarity of team objectives

- active participation–information sharing and influence over decision making

- task orientation

- support for innovation.

The leader cannot lead or influence team effectiveness without commitment and co-operation from the members. This will make a difference to team identity and their agreement to work together for a common purpose. Recruitment of a team leader requires the preparation of a job description and person specification. Defining the leadership qualities is an important aspect of this process and a few suggested items are listed in Box 6.3. The team leader can frequently be recruited from one of the existing team but there are occasions when the leadership skills do not exist. This has to be acknowledged and external candidates sought. Box 6.4 provides an example of a Team Leader job description.

Box 6.3 Leadership qualities.

■ Ability to motivate and generate enthusiasm.

■ Effective communicator – verbal and written.

■ Ability to facilitate and co-ordinate work.

■ Ability to consult and plan.

■ Ability to delegate appropriately.

■ A sense of humour.

Box 6.4 Specimen job description: Nurse Team Leader.

Hours   37½ hours per week

Grade   G

Qualifications   RGN with at least three years experience working in a primary care setting, preferably holding a community qualification. Management and teaching skills are an advantage.

Accountable to GP partnership

Job purpose   As leader of the nursing team you will be responsible for effective nursing care for the practice population.

Key areas of responsibility

Team leadership

■ Co-ordinate the activities of the nursing team.

■ Be responsible for the nursing team budget and provide regular reports.

Box 6.4 Continued

- Be responsible for appraising the nursing team members and encouraging individual professional development.

- Liaise with other members of the primary healthcare team to encourage communication on patient care and nursing team development.

- Represent the nursing team at practice policy development meetings.

- Develop and maintain a motivated and enthusiastic team.

Clinical care

- Be responsible for developing a practice profile to identify nursing needs.

- Develop a system of clinical audit which involves all members of the nursing team.

- Be responsible for the provision of nursing care to specific patient groups, e.g. chronic disease management, family planning.

- Be responsible for ensuring efficient recall systems are maintained.

- Be able to promote evidence-based care and change practice appropriately.

- Be competent to teach other nurses as necessary.

- Be responsible for developing and maintaining clinical guidelines, e.g. wound management, infection control, vaccine storage and usage.

- Maintain the UKCC *Code of Conduct* and *Scope of Professional Practice* standards.

- Abide by legal and statutory regulations.

Confidentiality

Much of the work relating to patients is confidential in nature and must not be communicated to other persons outside the group providing a duty of care.

Health and Safety at Work Act

It is the responsibility for all employees to comply with the requirements of the Act and to adhere to safe working practices.

Conditions of employment

To be specified by the practice.

Flexibility

Adjustments in responsibilities of the post may be required from time to time. Any adjustments will be made in consultation with the postholder.

The following process is recommended for selecting candidates:

- candidates should be invited to meet key practice personnel informally over coffee or lunch
- in the formal interview, candidates should be asked to do a presentation on a chosen topic for 10–15 minutes
- a schedule of interview questions should be used with each candidate which can be scored by the interview panel to ensure consistency.

As this is a post with clinical responsibility candidates should be asked to produce their professional portfolio at the interview. The scope of the team leader's job will have been determined in the job description and the levels of responsibility should be clear, particularly in relation to business planning and the assessment of health needs. The strategic issues will need to fit into the overall direction set by stakeholders such as the general practitioners and the health authority.

Conclusion

The titles and specialisms applicable to nurses working in the community are under review as part of proposals to rationalise the UKCC register. If the regulatory body for nursing makes it easier to organise integrated nursing teams in primary care, then the tentative changes seen so far will gather speed and confidence. This is not to say that the process is easy. The complexity of nursing roles should not be underestimated, but this should not be allowed to prevent the breaking down of traditional boundaries within a strategic framework of patient-centred care.

References

1 Roy S (1990) *Nursing in the Community: a report of the Working Group.* North West Thames Regional Health Authority, London.
2 Wiltshire FHSA (1993) *Nursing Roles in Primary Care.* Unpublished report.
3 Jansen PGM, Kenkstra A, Abu-Saad HH and Van der Zee J (1997) Differential practice and specialisation in community nursing: a descriptive study in the Netherlands. *Health Soc Care Comm.* 5(4):219–26.

4 UKCC (1992) *Scope of Professional Practice.* UKCC, London.
5 North Thames NHS Executive (1996) *The Development of Nursing and Health Visiting Roles in Clinical Practice.* NHSE, London.
6 West MA and Pillinger T (1996) *Team Building in Primary Healthcare: an evaluation.* Health Education Authority, London.

7
Integrated nursing teams: sprouting up everywhere?

Peter Hodder

'Given a clean start, nobody would create the structure and process of the current primary care team.'[1]

This chapter describes a number of integrated nursing teams (INTs) and demonstrates their application in primary care. It also provides a brief overview of the development of general practice and community nursing which demonstrates the significant differences between the two groups. The most notable of these is the power and influence general practitioners have compared with community nurses which both enables and hinders the development of INTs.

The hallmarks of general practice are accessibility, advice, diagnosis and treatment of illness. Its roots can be traced to the 19th century apothecaries but it was not until 1911, as part of the Liberal Government's social policy reforms, that the state provision of general medical care for low wage earners was proposed.[2] The *National Insurance Act* took two years to reach the Statute Book, largely due to the considerable opposition the Bill received from general practitioners. They were concerned that the State would take control of their work, diminish their autonomy as practitioners and reduce their income. They were persuaded to join the scheme only after they won concessions that ensured their independent status and secured financial remuneration based on the number of patients on a 'list'.

History repeated itself in 1946. The *National Health Service Act* met with opposition from the medical profession, this time mainly from the hospital doctors. In order to push the Act forward Aneurin Bevan conceded, and is said to have 'stuffed their mouths with gold'.[3] General practitioners maintained their independent practitioner status and continued on their pre-NHS path, separated from the mainstream of NHS policy and finance which, in turn, paid little attention to the place of primary care in the health system.[4] Over time general practitioners became the poor relation of the hospital specialist, yet steadfastly maintained their generalist skills. More recently the medical profession, with considerable misgivings, has been forced to accept legislation which pushed general practitioners into accepting the internal market, and in 1990 a new contract.[5,6]

The workload of general practitioners has reportedly increased considerably since the introduction of the 1990 Contract and the NHS reforms. Some feel demoralised, whilst others have been empowered to make significant changes on a local basis to the way care is provided.[7] Many initiatives have involved greater delegation of tasks to practice and community nurses. But should general practitioners relinquish some aspects of their role, encourage the 'substitution' trend and push work towards nurse practitioners within INTs?

The roots of community nursing can be traced back to the religious orders, parish nurses and poor law committees. It appears that health visiting started in Manchester when the Ladies' Sanitary Reform Association employed paid visitors to 'visit all and sundry, concentrating on cleanliness, good management and good living, helping the sick and advising mothers on the care of their children'.[8]

The first whole time staff appear to have been employed by the local authority in Buckinghamshire in 1892. Not until 1919 and the establishment of the Ministry of Health, was it deemed necessary to have qualifications to undertake such work. Although no formal training was required to become a midwife, health visitors were required to undertake a two-year training course which included training in the social sciences and domestic subjects. Formalised training for sick nurses and health visitors (who were also required to have midwifery experience) was imposed by the 1925 *Nurses Act*.

Twenty years later the contribution of community nurses was recognised in the *NHS Act* that required every local authority to make provision for health visiting and home nursing services. A mechanism of integration with general practitioners was not even considered, yet compared with the inherent resistance of the medical professions it is relatively easy to influence community nursing. Several Government reports have had significant impacts on service delivery.[9-12]

The contribution of community nursing has been increasingly recognised over the last hundred years. Indeed the present Government insists community nursing is to be part of the commissioning process within primary care groups.[13] What is unclear is who exactly will participate: nurses on the ground or their management directors?

Despite the potential of these recent developments, nurses have not, so far at least, enjoyed the same level of power and influence as general practitioners. They have never stood up, as a profession, and resisted legislation. Perhaps the time is approaching where the responsibility and accountability for planning and purchasing, albeit shared with others, will fundamentally change community nursing.

Primary healthcare teams

The term primary healthcare team (PHCT) first appeared in a government report in 1974.[14] It announced: 'The aim is to create a PHCT in which general practitioners, home nurses, health visitors and in some cases social workers and dentists, work together as an inter-disciplinary team, thus facilitating co-ordination and mutual support in the planning and delivery of care'. This is less a definition of the purpose of the primary care teams than an aspiration of what (if a *team* could be formed) it could achieve.

As much by accident as strategic planning, an opportunity arose for community nurses and general practitioners to be accommodated in 'health centres', built and managed by the local authorities. Considered to be cost-effective accommodation, some general practitioners found themselves housed in the same building as the community nurses, who by and large were worked to geographically defined areas, rather than to the general practitioner's practice list population.

A Royal Commission saw the centres as 'proper premises for general practitioners, with good equipment and well organised staff' and part of a 'continuing process' in which eventually all general practitioners and the local health authority staff would be linked together to form a single team.[15] No recommendations were given on *how* they would become a team, and it seemed that the Commission thought this would be an inevitable development of general practitioners and community nurses being housed under one roof. Some general practitioners were suspicious and reluctant to work with nurses who (at that time) were local authority employed staff. General practitioners who saw an opportunity to develop teamwork and preventative medicine were accused by their colleagues of 'dismantling their empires'.[16]

In the 1980s policy makers began to pay increasing attention to primary care. The rising costs of healthcare, demographic trends and changing patterns of illness led to an emphasis on preventative measures that could be provided more economically outside hospitals.[17,18] By the late 1990s, this has been translated into a new emphasis on locality-based commissioning, led by primary care. Current thinking suggests that primary care services should be 'focused on the general practice population'.[19] How do INTs fit into this evolving policy framework?

Nursing teams

The difficulties of delivering a service and creating a team in primary care were discussed in the Cumberlege Report, commissioned by the Secretary of State for Health.[10] The problems of 'attachment', where the nurse works to a geographically defined area and not to the practice list population, were highlighted. Cumberlege found that teamwork was 'fractured and piecemeal'.[20] Community nurses felt torn between two different organisations, separated from each other and from other specialist nurses and resulting in their roles becoming traditional and set. As a remedy, the Report recommended that 'neighbourhood nursing teams' (NNTs) be developed with nurses brought together in teams to facilitate effective collaboration between 'all' community health workers. This is an important feature of what INTs are attempting to achieve today, but in an entirely different policy context. The Report recognised the structural difficulties associated with health authority employees and general practitioner employees, referring specifically to practice nurses. It recommended one structure be formed – practice nurses should be transferred to the employment (and management) of health authorities.

Focusing on the clinical competency of community nurses, the Report proposed the development of nurse prescribing and the role of nurse practitioners. These two concepts are making slow but gradual progress within the overall structure of integrated nursing in primary care.

Nurses welcomed the Cumberlege Report, largely because it recognised their professional status and the contribution they could make in community health. Contracts with general practitioners were recommended that would stipulate the aims of the NNTs, the frequency of meetings with general practitioners and referral protocols between the two groups. These were important elements in establishing a base on which to build a functioning service. Some INTs have, as will be shown later, discussed these issues both formally (by external facilitation) and informally through joint meetings.

Primary care teamwork: fact or fiction?

Prominent reports over the last 25 years have highlighted the importance of teamwork in primary care. Apart from Roy, none actually contained any approaches which aimed to improve teamwork. The reports recognised that many on the ground had attempted to work with each other, but clearly working 'with each other' does not constitute teamwork. This is an important lesson for INTs which may yet struggle like the proposed NNTs and 'primary care teams' before them.

Community nurses work to policies and procedures established by their community trust organisations. Very often, priorities are set for them. Such procedures, policies and priorities may not be compatible with those of general practitioners and such variances are significant barriers to teamwork. Elwyn and Øvretveit have discussed these obstacles in further depth in Chapter 4 and they have been recognised by many commentators over the last 20 years.[21,22] Beales for example refers to 'the uneasy alliance of people ultimately devoted to different and frequently opposing sides'.[23] Yet in spite of these observations, there has been no suggestion on a national level that policies or structures need attention.

Implementation of policies and procedures, funding issues, maintenance of community trust services mean that, in spite of admirable intentions, management 'by interference' is felt to operate at all levels within primary care. The Community Trust ultimately 'own' the nurses and this allows the management to arbitrarily move staff from one area to another without regard for the professional relationships developed between staff and patients. Based on the system of the general practitioner who 'shouts the loudest gets what s/he wants' an inequality of service provision occurs and allows a frustrated, often fragmented group to operate an unco-ordinated service.

The contracting process between fundholding general practitioners and community trusts has offered some (temporary) stability, but the new arrangement for locality-based commissioning is likely to change this relationship once again. All the INTs cited here are working with large fundholding practices. Are we merely seeing powerful general practitioners exert their powers or are INTs bottom-up initiatives, led by nurses who want to improve the services they can offer within their nursing practice?[24]

Developing teamwork in primary care is hindered by the structural and professional differences between general practitioners and community nurses. Is the development of INTs merely a short-term and inadequate solution to a long-term problem, seized upon by frustrated doctors and forward thinking nurses? Perhaps so. Let's turn our attention to a few of the INTs that have developed in the UK.

Examples of integrated nursing teams

This account of INTs is based on observation and discussion – it is not based on in-depth research, neither is it a comprehensive survey of all the developments known to be taking place. Nevertheless, the examples provided give, I hope, a flavour of the current forces operating within the development of primary care organisations. Three models of INTs appear to be emerging: the self-managed teams, specific practice focus teams (rather like the traditional attachment) and seconded teams. All have a number of common themes, namely:

- the development of joint working between practice, district nurses and health visitors, which allows tasks to be shared

- closer liaison with general practitioners and other primary care staff with a recognition of each other's roles in the care of patients

- development of the nursing profession

- an attempt to bridge the structural gap between community nurses and general practitioners.

Different models are developing at different rates and include different professional groups. Again they appear to be operating at three levels.

1 Primary level – offering basic care within the practice and to the practice population.

2 Specialist primary care level – working to a mutually agreed set of standards/protocols that involve all members of the team that work with the defined practice population.

3 Shared primary care level – recognises that other general practitioners/ nurses outside the practice have specialist skills to offer certain patient groups who can be referred, thus allowing shared care. In its embryonic form, this example is best seen among the larger multifunds and commissioning groups, particularly in Birmingham.

All of the case histories cited fall into the first two levels. Most INTs focus on the district nurses, health visitors and practice nurses.

Thornton Medical Centre

Clearly, for the Thornton Medical Centre in Lancashire their existing 'nurse attachment' was unsatisfactory. Led by a general practitioner, the nurses developed an integrated approach to care that, over a relatively short period of time, improved the morale, working practices and efficiency of the team.[25] Operating from a health centre, the same group of workers only came together through the process of integration, stability and ownership – three important components of teamwork. Increased integration was partly achieved by re-organising the practice accommodation and the up-take of services. The district nurses and health visitors moved into shared offices and the treatment room was shared between the practice nurses and the community staff. 'Misuse of services' was curtailed because in the new arrangements the community nurses could recognise the unnecessary duplication of effort and felt able to change the system.[25] Individuals were encouraged to contribute ideas and simple but effective modifications were implemented. Policy issues were not addressed initially but referrals between the nurses were streamlined.

The Winch Lane Surgery

The Thornton practice was mirrored in a very different way by the Winch Lane Surgery in Haverfordwest.[26] Both attempted to reduce management 'interference' by creating team co-ordinator roles within the INT, although in both cases the local community trusts played active parts in the process.

The INT at Winch Lane was developed by a general practitioner that wanted to achieve more effective teamwork. Inspired by the process of acting as a mentor to the practice nurse, the general practitioner discussed the potential of an INT with his medical colleagues and his local health authority. The facilitation offered by the Dyfed Powys Health Authority encouraged debate and the open involvement of the local community trust. The team devised strategies to deal with the day-to-day issues: a form of 'operational policy'. The development of shared protocols enhanced team-work through the acceptance of mutually accepted responsibilities.

Llyn y fran Practice

The development of the INT in Llyn y fran (Cardiganshire, mid-Wales) is a good example of general practitioners setting the direction for the nursing professions. The practice joined other local surgeries in the area to participate in a local/general practitioner commissioning pilot.

The community nurses were invited on a 'teambuilding' exercise together with all other clinical and administrative staff within the practice.

The general practitioners played an active part in the exercise which was organised by a Director of Training from one of the local Community Trusts. In parallel with the Thornton and Winch Lane initiatives, a team co-ordinator was appointed.

The nurses were left with many unanswered questions. Would there be a change of employment status? What changes would there be to role responsibilities and professional accountabilities? What local management arrangements would be in place? These concerns are commonplace and a symptom of the fractured arrangements in place for the employment of 'practice' and 'community' staff. Without the level of team facilitation evident elsewhere, the Llyn y fran INT has developed more slowly but their willingness to try new ways of working, coupled with a desire to expand and improve services for patients in a wide rural area, is clearly evident.

Premier Healthcare Trust

Premier Health, a community healthcare trust in South Staffordshire, led the way in devolving budget responsibility to local groups of nurses, known as 'self-managed teams.' Through their Primary Care Unit, the nursing teams are offered a great deal of support. Working in conjunction with John Moores University, Liverpool, an in-depth professional development portfolio has been developed. The nurses are encouraged to attend skill building sessions open to both practice nurses and other healthcare professionals including general practitioners. In the early days of fundholding, this strategic initiative allowed Premier Health to provide services for general practitioner fundholders in other regions, the first being in Cheshire. Others followed, including practices as far away as the Four Elms Medical Centre in Cardiff and a practice in Monmouth, Gwent, clearly demonstrating the enthusiasm of those with their hands on the levers of change to see new arrangements in place for primary care nursing. Oxford (see Chapter 8) and Walsall have also adopted this model of devolved nursing budgets. Both areas offered self-managed team guidance, support and facilitation.

Tile Hill

Eight general practitioners in Tile Hill, Coventry, secured total separation from the community trust management by formally seconding nursing staff to their substantive general practitioner managed service. In reality, the Tile Hill general practitioners were a pilot site that preceded fund-holding consortia. They formed a management board chaired by a lead general practitioner. Following informal interviews, community nurses were seconded thus ensuring stability, integration and ownership. In essence the community nurses interviewed the general practitioner and team manager. To ensure that prospective secondees understood the process, a representative from their community trust was present. Safeguards were provided to the secondee so that their employment, terms and conditions of service did not change.

The pilot was extremely successful and the service became substantive in 1993, appointing a team co-ordinator to manage the service on a day-to-day basis. A district nurse and health visitor take this post in rotation on a six-monthly basis. The team manages to co-operate well, similar to the experiences reported from Winch Lane and Thornton. Working to a set of agreed policies and procedures, change was managed in a positive way. Communication between team members was improved and patients reported a high level of satisfaction.[27] Financial savings were re-invested enabling the team to expand its range of primary care services.[28]

A second general practitioner-managed primary care team was formed three years later in the Hillfields area of Coventry. The secondment process was the same as that for Tile Hill, and the team identity quickly formed. Tile Hill and Hillfields believe that 'secondment' has overcome some of the organisational issues that can so easily get in the way of effective team-work, although the practice nurses have not been integrated to the same extent as at Winch Lane and Thornton.

However, the general practitioners in both teams have not, to date, wanted to fully integrate practice nurses. Secondment worked for Tile Hill and Hillfields because local doctors agreed to work together and 'pool' their community nursing resources. Each site has around 20 000 patients and a sufficient number of community nurses were seconded to ensure the teams could absorb their own cover/leave arrangements.

Conclusion

INTs are 'sprouting up' everywhere or at least the push to 'integrate' the nurses who work at the sharp end of primary care now seems irresistible. The missing component is the policy and structural framework to make it happen. Achieving integration, stability and ownership and eradicating or minimising management by interference are important steps towards effective teamwork. But if the patients and clients are to truly benefit, integration needs to be multidisciplinary and valued by all the professions. Where, for example, do community psychiatric nurses, midwives and physiotherapists fit into an INT? Are they part of it or do they link into it? Is the general practitioner part of the INT or is it simply a nursing organisation?

Community nurses and social services will, it seems, have a greater involvement in the commissioning of care. There may be greater opportunities for nurses to contribute to the shape of healthcare within local communities and share in the balance of power. Whether integrated nursing teams represent a wise step in the direction of co-ordinated healthcare, only time will tell.

References

1 Pringle M (1992) The developing primary care partnership. *BMJ*. **305**: 624–6.
2 Fry J (1988) *General Practice and Primary Healthcare 1940–80*. Nuffield Provincial Hospitals Trust, London.
3 Abel-Smith B (1964) *The Hospitals 1800–1948*. Heinemann, Oxford. *See also* Ham C (1985) *Health Policy in Britain: the policy and organisation of the National Health Service* (2nd ed). Macmillan, London.
4 Gordon P and Pampling D (1996) Primary healthcare: its characteristics and potential. In: P Gordon and J Hadley (eds) *Extending Primary Care: polyclinics, resource centres, hospital-at-home*. Radcliffe Medical Press, Oxford.
5 Department of Health (1990) *National Health Service and Community Care Act 1990*. HMSO, London.
6 Department of Health and The Welsh Office (1989) *General Practice in the National Health Service: a new contract*. HMSO, London.
7 Exworth M (1996) Power points. *Health Service J*. **106**:24–5.
8 Ham C (1985) *Health Policy in Britain: the policy and organisation of the National Health Service* (2nd ed). Macmillan, London.
9 Briggs A (1972) *Report of the Committee on Nursing*. DHSS, Scottish Home and Health Department and Welsh Office, London.
10 Cumberlege Department of Health and Social Security (1986) *Neighbourhood Nursing: a focus for care. Report of the Community Nursing Review Team*. HMSO, London.
11 Griffiths R (1988) *Community Care: agenda for action. A Report to the Secretary of State for Social Services*. HMSO, London.
12 Roy S (1990) *Nursing in the Community. A Report of the Working Group*. North West Thames Regional Health Authority, London.

13 Department of Health (1997) *The New NHS: modern, dependable.* The Stationery Office, London.

14 Harding W (1981) *Report of the Joint Working Group on Primary Healthcare Teams. Standing Medical Advisory Committee and Midwifery Advisory Committee.* HMSO, London.

15 Todd A (1968) *Royal Commission on Medical Education Report.* HMSO, London.

16 Hasler J (1993) The primary healthcare team: history and contractual farces. In: M Pringle (ed) *Change and Teamwork in Primary Care.* BMJ Publishing Group, London.

17 Allsop J (1990) *Changing Primary Care: the role of facilitators.* King's Fund Centre, London.

18 Taylor D (1991) *Developing Primary Care: opportunities for the 1990s. Research Report 10.* King's Fund Institute and the Nuffield Provincial Hospitals Trust, London.

19 NHS Management Executive (1993) *New World, New Opportunities: nursing in primary healthcare.* HMSO, London.

20 Rogers R (1986) *Neighbourhood Nursing. Report of a Conference.* Report No KFC 86/127. King's Fund, London.

21 Grieg D (1988) *Teamwork in General Practice.* Castle House Publications, London.

22 Salisbury C (1991) Working in partnership with nurses. *British J Gen Prac.* **41**:398–9.

23 Beales J (1978) *Sick Health Centres and How to Make Them Better.* Pitman Medical Publishing, London.

24 Paterson J (1997) Stage II set for new nursing teams. *Practice Nurse.* **14**: 425–8.

25 Richardson S (1997) Integrated approach is a success. *GP.* **Jan** 3:33.

26 Jones R (1997) *Integrated Nursing Team Project.* Unpublished report to Dyfed Powys Health Authority.

27 Coventry Family Health Services Authority (1993) *Annual Report.* Coventry FHSA, Coventry.

28 Hodder P (1995) Towards an integrated primary healthcare team. *Value for Money Update (NHS Executive)* **1**:6–7.

8

Budgets and management: the Oxfordshire approach

Lisa Whordley and Jane Dauncey

The development of 'self-management' is an important part of the process of achieving effective integrated nursing teams (INTs). It is, however, inevitable that the issues of accountability and risk become prime concerns when devolving management and budgetary responsibility. In this chapter strategies to manage these risks will be discussed and the benefits identified and explored. The approach in Oxfordshire has been developmental and, from the start, efforts have been made to learn from the experiences of others. However, there is very little written on this subject and much of the work has evolved as issues have been addressed. This work is therefore based on the experiences in Oxfordshire between 1994 and 1998.

In 1994, the health authority and GP fundholders, as the main purchasers of the Trust's services, decided to change their specification for the purchasing of community nursing services to one that focused on the formation of INTs, with decision making taking place as close to the patient as possible. There were three major reasons for this policy change.

The first was to improve the service to patients, making sure that decisions made about their care were made within the primary healthcare team (PHCT). Prior to this, decisions relating to the use of resources by community nurses was performed externally by nurse managers. The second reason was to improve the integration of care provided by district nurses, practice nurses and health visitors by reducing overlaps and by trying to break down the traditional professional barriers. The third objective was to reduce management costs by removing the tier of community nurse management. The money released was re-invested in the clinical nursing service. For community trusts, with community nursing income known in advance because of the contracting arrangements, the main imperative was to exert a downward pressure on management overheads.[1]

To achieve these objectives, the Oxfordshire Community Health NHS Trust decided to devolve management and budgetary responsibilities to the community nursing team. Every team would have the ability to make its own decisions about the services provided, and have the responsibility for the resources allocated to them. The principles of the changes conformed with the Trust's strategy of empowering staff by devolving responsibility to those delivering nursing care. The empowerment strategy aimed to equip all staff to make decisions and required a flat management structure. Although the Trust recognised that this was an ambitious venture, it was implemented simultaneously in all 88 community nursing teams over a short period of time starting in April 1995.

It was decided, with the purchasers, that 'self-managing' teams of G grade nurses did not each require a team leader. It was agreed that district nurses and health visitors should, by virtue of their education and training, have all the core skills needed for teamworking. It was recognised, however, that they would need training to acquire the management skills and, in some cases, leadership competencies and that certain tasks required a named individual to accept overall accountability. Teams could not be given a devolved budget until an accountable person was appointed and trained. Other responsibilities of the self-managing team were to be taken on by nurses with the most appropriate skills. This may relate to a clinical area, e.g. devising a strategy for accident prevention or wound care, or a nurse could accept responsibility for a personnel function, e.g. managing a skill-mix review. Before the changes, many G grade community nurses, anticipating the process, had already accepted these new management responsibilities.

Both the Trust, the health authority and GP fundholders were keen to avoid creating another management tier. The objective was to integrate the three main nursing disciplines – district nursing, practice nursing and health visiting – whilst accepting the tensions created by having dual employment arrangements. It was judged that the self-managing concept would be more effective than the rigid imposition of a team leader structure. Nevertheless, many teams elected a chair to take a co-ordination role.

To facilitate the teams it was agreed that the Trust would employ primary care development nurses with specific management and leadership skills. They have been critical to the success of the self-management process. Working with their colleagues in the finance and personnel directorates, they have implemented processes to manage risk and have identified training needs. This has led to a supportive framework for the community nursing teams. Another aspect of the role has been the responsibility to encourage clinical development and to ensure that innovations are shared between teams. This has led to interdisciplinary work with GPs, and is resulting in the development of strategies and protocols that are widely applicable.

The key issues identified were the management of the change process, education and training and the resolution of concerns about risk and accountability. Tensions were experienced about these two latter areas that have taken considerable time and negotiation to resolve. The removal of the community nurse manager role was implemented extremely rapidly in the 88 teams, and caused stress and confusion for both the community nurses and the Trust. As it was a purchasing decision, the nurses on the ground had not been consulted. Some of the nurses embraced the self-management concept without recognising the added competencies required, and increased the risks for both themselves and the Trust. Others, however, found it very stressful and were frightened by the potential risks. This again emphasises the need to provide education and support when developing processes that change long established working relationships.

To help fill the gap identified by the Trust in 1995, a manual of procedures and protocols was produced to provide information for effective decision making and risk management. This manual was rejected by a substantial number of teams – it was considered as an 'interference' and an attempt by the Trust to be 'controlling'. This was symptomatic of the split loyalties experienced by many community nurses who seem to belong to two organisations, seemingly pulling in different directions. It also highlighted the difficulties that GPs, practice managers and nurses experience in understanding the Trust's accountability and risk management issues. Expressions such as 'risk averse', 'controlling' and 'unwilling to change' were applied to the Trust and hindered the development of an accountability framework. The result effect of all this was to increase the stress experienced by the community nurses who were struggling to cope with new management responsibilities.

The Trust also had limited understanding of the GMS regulations and practice and fund management responsibilities and there was little opportunity to resolve these problems. Some of the misunderstandings related to the differences between the different legal responsibilities of a GP practice as a small employer and a NHS Trust as a much larger organisation.

The Trust had to ensure that clinical practice was as safe and that the management of risk was robust. As this need became more widely recognised within the primary care system in Oxfordshire a new accountability framework was implemented. This provides a structure that helps manage risk – both to individuals as employees and the Trust as an employer. The response from teams has been positive and demonstrates the processes needed to support self-managing teams. The framework contains five sections:

1 Clinical

2 Personnel

3 Finance

4 Information

5 Health and safety.

Funding INTs

It has often been said that one of the major obstacles to achieving fully integrated nursing teams is the existence of two separate funding streams and, in most cases, two separate employers of community nurses and practice nurses. In 1996, the official document *Primary Care: delivering the future*, went so far as to state that 'the existing legal framework can act as a barrier to progress'.[2] Community nurses are funded through Hospital and Community Health Services (HCHS) allocations. Practice nursing, by comparison, is funded entirely separately via the General Medical Services (GMS) fund. Historically, practice nurses have been funded along with other practice staff on a reimbursement basis. Until recently there has been little scope for the amalgamation of practice nurse and community nursing budgets unless, as in some areas of the country, the practice nurses are employed through a community trust.

Devolving the community nursing budget

The process of devolving the community nursing budget to local teams has been increasingly adopted by community trusts around the country to varying degrees over the last five years. Trusts that have chosen to devolve their budgets to a team level have met two major difficulties. First, the historic underfunding of community nursing budgets becomes transparent. Many trusts set budgets on the basis of a 'vacancy factor' being available within the year to offset the lack of income (*see* Box 8.1). This 'vacancy factor' is the slippage money which results as a result of the time gap between a nurse leaving and a new nurse coming into post, hence the name. It became common practice to delay recruiting for a month or

Box 8.1   Dr White and partners community nursing budget allocation 1995/96.

	£
Income	177 884
Salaries	
District nursing	98 650
Health visiting	45 789
Clerical	11 124
Agency staff	3651
Non-pay	
Travel	18 746
Uniforms	1120
Consumables and continence	3231
Administration	2145
Vacancy factor	−6572

two in order to bring budgets back into balance – a bone of contention with many GP fundholders, who felt strongly that it was unethical and exploitative. Trusts have only been able to devolve what was 'historically' available. This has once again served to illustrate the lack of funding for this service. In the absence of an objective standard of nursing 'adequacy', the aim must be to provide the best possible service within the limits of available resources.[3]

The second major issue is that of equity. The service must ensure that the range and quality of services does not vary significantly across the county or between patient groups.[4] Many trusts have examined the relative funding available for community nursing, either on a practice or locality basis, e.g. an equity exercise. An equity formula has then been applied to determine whether a practice is relatively under- or overfunded compared with others. The difficult task is to decide which teams gain and lose resources – a process complicated by GP fundholding practices who are unwilling to have their allocations altered. In fact, many GPs choose to invest fundholding savings, or 'growth' money, into community nursing and this adds to the imbalance within the system. Every equity formula yet devised is viewed as flawed by some stakeholders and none, as yet, have included a measure of what is adequate or efficient.

In Oxfordshire, budgets have been devolved to teams apart from some items 'blocked back' by mutual agreement, to be managed centrally by the Trust (*see* Box 8.2). These items are Trust overheads, continence products and contributions to an equipment library. Further thought is now being given to other high cost items such as enteral feeding products. Most items were devolved on a historic spend basis (where information was available at team level). The remaining items such as continence products and equipment were devolved on a rough capitation basis.

Box 8.2   Dr Green and partners community nursing allocation 1997/98.

	£
Income	152 171
Salaries	
District nursing	78 621
Health visiting	36 756
Clerical	5002
Agency staff	1214
Non-pay	
Travel	6783
Uniforms	983
Consumables and continence	1875
Administration	1516
Premises rental	2030
Service charges	750
Equipment	130
Telephones	43
Contributions to central services	
Trust overheads	15 080
Continence products for children with special needs	732
Equipment library contributions	267

How are decisions made?

An essential part of the Oxfordshire model has been that community nurses manage their own budget. This requires a named person to assume responsibility for managing the budget on a day-to-day basis and it is important that there are support mechanisms in place to advise as necessary. To this end, finance workshops are run in a different locality each month and, where necessary, advice may be sought from the Trust finance team or primary care development nurse. The accountants working in primary care are encouraged to visit the teams in their own bases wherever possible and meetings are available on request.

Sickness and maternity leave cover

In the first instance, teams tended to retreat and cut ties with many other practices that they may have worked with quite closely in the past. This was very noticeable when it came to covering for sickness and maternity leave cover. Most localities had cover arrangements in place which, by and large, were discarded as people attempted to work in self-contained units. This inevitably led to problems, either a lack of cover or overspends on bank staff. Some salary budgets also began to look overspent as payments for enhanced hours, not previously incurred, began to appear. However, teams which at first needed to break away from the way in which they traditionally worked, have realised that, from time to time, it makes sense to work as part of a wider co-operative.

Are devolved budgets cost effective?

The results suggest that the system is cost effective in that there appear to be persistent underspends across most budgets. These are made up partly through good housekeeping and partly because of delays, or inability, to recruit staff. There are, however, many hidden support costs and increased transaction costs for trusts. The mechanics of communicating with 88 teams on an individual basis rather than via a network of senior nurses has cost implications even in the simplest terms, i.e. photocopying and postage. The new system led to increased numbers of staff working in the finance and personnel functions to answer the greater number of enquiries. It is also an indisputable fact that levels of stress increased considerably, both within the Trust and community staff. Individuals had very little time to adjust and prepare for the new systems, again reflected in the sickness absence costs that can be attributed to the changes.

Accountability

An accountability framework should establish exactly what is meant by freedom to 'manage the budget'. Trust staff are required to observe standing financial instructions and this is equally applicable to the named and accountable team budget holder. Adhering to the financial protocols of the Trust may at times cause friction at the practice level where there is a culture of less formal mechanisms for financial management.

Conclusion

Community nurses in Oxfordshire have been on a journey towards the achievement of self-managing teams for nearly three years and have achieved a great deal. There has been better and more effective use of resources. Teams have more ownership of the issues facing community nursing, and have become more active and vocal in finding solutions. There is local decision making by empowered practitioners. As with any upheaval, there have been expressions of stress and concerns about pressure on clinical time. Nevertheless, the auditors are happy that the Trust has effectively managed the risk associated with the development of 'self-managed' nursing teams.

The main obstacles continue to be associated with the two separate streams of funding and the marked cultural differences between the 'empowered' culture of the Trust and the more traditional structure of general practice. There are disadvantages to adopting devolved budgets. Many of them centre around the fact that they are not sufficiently large to accommodate any degree of financial risk, such as, for example, extended sickness cover, patients requiring expensive consumables or for even the most basic aspects such as managing incremental drift. We have also struggled to find an acceptable way in which to manage year-end balances. Most teams have year-end underspends which they naturally wish to carry forward to the next financial year. Some teams have overspends, largely through external factors of no fault of their own. The Trust is required to meet external finance limits and does not have a mechanism for assisting overspent teams. A clear outcome of having devolved budgets is that teams work very hard to manage their budgets effectively, and therefore feel strong ownership of any accrued savings. Fundholding has also muddied the waters and every year-end to date we have entered into a 'whose money is it anyway' debate.

The majority of GPs supported the changes and have continued to do so. One of the benefits is the wider understanding by GPs of the Trust's support services, its expertise and its economies of scale. This has led to some opening discussions about the development of a Primary Care Trust. Few could have predicted that by 1999 primary care groups (PCGs) would be formed with community nurses taking an important role alongside their GP colleagues. The experiences and skills gained by the self-management process have given us an excellent start. PCGs should be able to take responsibility for a single unified budget covering most aspects of care and get the best fit between resources and need. The changes in financial arrangements will overcome the difficulties created by having two separate streams of money and will inevitably involve closer working ties between practices and between nursing teams. None of this will be an easy task but the foundations of an integrated primary care service have been laid. Now we all need to build on them.

References

1 Audit Commission (1996) *What the Doctor Ordered.* Audit Commission, London.
2 Department of Health (1996) *Primary Care: delivering the future.* HMSO, London.
3 Department of Health (1996) *A Service with Ambition.* HMSO, London.
4 Department of Health (1997) *The New NHS: modern, dependable.* The Stationery Office, London.

9

The legal aspects

Bridgit Dimond

The establishment of integrated nursing teams (INTs) in primary care has not resulted from any specific laws. A vast range of laws, both statutory and judge-made, apply to the teams that work in primary care.

Introduction: brief introduction to the legal system

Our laws derive from two main sources: statutory law, i.e. Acts of Parliament, and the common law, i.e. judge-made or case law. The law that relates to the subject of this book derives from both sources. There is no legislation that covers team functioning, merely a jigsaw of different Acts of Parliament and legal principles declared by the courts which apply to the range of potential legal issues which arise.

Once enacted the *Human Rights Bill 1997* will enable individuals who consider that their rights (as set out in the European Convention) have been infringed by a public authority to seek redress directly in the courts in the UK, rather than take the case to Strasbourg as at present. The implications of public authorities having to comply with the Convention may be extremely significant and costly.

Statutory framework and primary healthcare

The main statutes which apply to primary healthcare are noted in Box 9.1. These Acts define the duties of the Secretary of State and health authorities in relation to the provision of primary healthcare and also set out the management arrangements. The *NHS and Community Care Act 1990* created the internal market, defining purchasers and providers and establishing arrangements for GPs to become fundholders, purchasing services for their patients. The *National Health Service (Primary Care) Act 1997*, allows the introduction of new arrangements for the organisation and provision of primary healthcare. The recent White Paper proposes major changes to the organisation of health service provision which includes the abolition of the internal market within the NHS and the development of primary care groups which may become free-standing Primary Care Trusts.[1] The White Paper in Wales envisages local health groups that will agree long-term service agreements with local providers to meet the health needs of the population.[2]

Box 9.1   Statutes applying to primary healthcare.

■ *National Health Service Act 1977*

■ *National Health Service and Community Care Act 1990*

■ *National Health Service (Primary Care) Act 1997*

■ *NHS Act (1998 or 1999) following the 1997 White Paper on the NHS*

Team liability

The Court of Appeal in the Wilsher case stated clearly that the law does not recognise team liability.[3] Each individual member of the team is personally and professionally accountable for his or her own actions. Nor is it any defence to argue that a junior member of a team had carried out the work negligently, if the work should have been done by a senior member. The team itself has no legal significance. Some members of the team may however have a management responsibility for the functioning of the team – ensuring that the appropriate training has been given, taking administrative responsibility for team meetings, secretarial support, and also some responsibilities in relation to communications. Failures in fulfilling these responsibilities could lead to disciplinary or professional conduct proceedings. For example, if a nurse acted as the team leader she may have responsibilities for convening meetings, for checking that all the team members had received relevant communications and for ensuring that individual responsibilities were clearly identified. If she were to fail in carrying out these management functions and as a result harm befell a patient she could be held to account for these failings.

Individual accountability

It is therefore no defence, if harm has occurred as a result of his/her actions, for a team member to say 'I was obeying the instructions of the team'. The team member is personally and professionally accountable for his/her actions. This means that there could be liability in professional conduct proceedings and there could even be criminal prosecution and/or disciplinary proceedings as a result of breaches in the contract of employment. Civil action could also be brought against the employer for its vicarious liability for the negligence of an employee. If the team member is a self-employed professional then he or she would have to face personal civil action in the event of negligence causing harm. GPs, fundholder GPs and NHS Trusts may all be employers of team members and would therefore be vicariously liable for the negligence of their own employees. To establish vicarious liability it must be shown that the employee was negligent whilst acting in the course of employment. If the team member is a volunteer then he or she may be well advised to obtain insurance cover for any legal proceedings that arise from the voluntary work. Personal insurance may not be necessary if the volunteer is appointed and covered by a voluntary organisation.

Key workers

It follows from the absence of any team liability that if a member of the team is designated as a key worker, then that individual must ensure that he or she works within the limits of competence. Any expanded activities must only be carried out if the individual has the experience, knowledge and competence to perform them safely. This may mean that an individual has to be prepared to state clearly to the team that a particular activity which he or she is expected to undertake is outside his or her field of competence. This may take considerable courage. For example, a practice nurse may be designated as a patient's key worker, but if that individual needs the assistance of an experienced stoma nurse, then a specialist nurse should be brought in to assist the patient.

Scope of professional practice

The UKCC's guidance on expanding the role of the nurse can provide the framework within which an individual practitioner can develop her expertise. This would enable a key worker to become competent to carry out a much wider range of activities, thereby enabling the roles of several different professionals to be undertaken by a key worker. Through the acceptance of the six main principles of the Scope, a nurse could develop expertise in areas now covered by professions supplementary to medicine as well as other specialist fields of nursing practice. However, the individual involved has the legal responsibility to ensure competence in these new areas.

At present the legislation establishing the UKCC and its functions is under review.[4] The consultation paper issued by JM Consulting suggests that health visitors should no longer be separately registered on the UKCC register, and that post-registration qualifications and specialist training should be recorded but not as part of the UKCC register. The Government has accepted other similar recommendations and if the above proposal is supported, it will be easier to develop post-registration roles and responsibilities.

Nurse prescribing

District nurses and health visitors can, if they have completed the necessary additional training, be recognised as nurse prescribers. This has been made possible by the amending legislation that took place in 1992.[5] At present practice nurses who do not have district nursing or health visiting qualifications, are not able to become prescribers. This distinction between different members of the primary care nursing team is not justifiable and may well be removed in future amending legislation.

Nurse prescribers can only prescribe from a limited range of products set out in the *Nurses' Formulary*.[6] They would be personally responsible for any prescribing errors. Their employers would of course be vicariously liable for their action. Extending the role of the nurse by allowing restricted and supervised prescribing is clearly a key issue for the way in which primary care develops and the legal issues are crucial.[7]

Training and professional development

Whatever the designation of the nurse member of the primary care team, it is essential that they each receive the necessary training and professional development. This is of course a statutory requirement under PREP. However, team members have different terms of employment and in some cases the employer pays the full costs of education and training, including time off work and associated expenses. Others are expected to fund their own study leave and may use annual leave. The extent to which employees have a right to receive professional development at the employer's expense is unclear. Certainly the employer has a duty to ensure that staff are competent and a breach of this duty which led to harm could result in successful legal claims. However, the funding of such development is usually a matter for collective bargaining and part of the negotiations on the terms of service. It is clear that the shortage of nurses, particularly in some specialist areas, will compel employers to provide more favourable conditions for study leave and expenses.

Delegation and supervision

Where a senior health professional in a team delegates specific work to another professional, there could be liability if that delegation was inappropriate or the level of supervision inadequate. There would also be liability on the person accepting the delegated activity if there was an awareness that the task was outside the scope of competence. In other words, in order to be responsible for the actions of a junior, the senior must be personally at fault as a result of inappropriate delegation or supervision. There is no principle in English law that a superior is vicariously liable for the actions of a junior. The concept of vicarious liability only applies to the employer.

Managerial control and hierarchy

The fact that the team members do not have a single employer can frustrate any attempt to set up line management responsibilities within the team and can easily became a cause of conflict. What if the senior manager is not a member of the team and yet is giving instructions at variance to decisions taken within the organisation? For example, a district nurse, although managed by a nursing officer who holds a senior Trust position, may find that she has policies imposed (e.g. not to collect medicines from the local pharmacy for her clients) which are in conflict with duties expected of her by the team. Such potential conflicts need to be resolved before the professional becomes a member of the primary care team: it may well be necessary for external line managers to accept a curtailment of their authority.

Employment conditions

Many team members work for different employment agencies (social services, general practice, NHS Trust and voluntary organisations) and find that the conditions vary markedly. A social worker might have a case list ceiling of 25–30 clients, a psychiatric nurse might be expected to provide cover for 50 clients, a practice nurse might have a working week of 40 hours and a district nurse one of 37½ hours with flexible days-off as an added perk. Such differences, whilst not impossible to overcome, can potentially cause tensions and bitterness.[8]

Communication issues

There can be liability in law for failure to ensure effective communication. Good communication should theoretically be made easier as a result of 'integrating' nursing teams, but this will depend on having effective systems in place. Roles and responsibilities will need clarification and documentation will need to meet a high standard, preferably by allowing multiprofessional access to an integrated electronic information service. A failure of an individual to ensure effective communication with others, if this leads to patient harm, can result in a claim for negligence against the employer. If a district nurse failed to make sure that the GP was notified of a patient's deterioration, and harm occurred as a consequence, the failure to communicate could be the basis of an action for negligence.

Concept of self-managing teams

If the various employing authorities are prepared to delegate both the budget and the associated responsibilities then the team can make considerable progress, but it is essential that this process be monitored by the parent organisations. There is also a concept known as 'self-governance' that encourages professionals to accept the responsibility for their own actions.[9] Self-governance calls for all team members to 'own' their decisions, to manage their own work and build relationships and achieve desirable outcomes. The principles of partnership, equity, accountability and owner-ship apply to every person in the organisation. Since the concept is essentially horizontal, there is no place for hierarchical relationships in shared governance. There is considerable scope for the development of self-governance in integrated primary healthcare teams, but this will only take place if the organisations and senior management facilitate the necessary autonomy.

The team would find it difficult to work effectively if it did not have clearly identified resources. This requires employers to delegate appropriate budgets to meet team responsibilities. The power to vire funds between different compartments is important, as is a policy about what should happen to any savings. Responsibility for the control of this expenditure cannot rest with an ill-defined team but must be made the responsibility of a budget holder.

Status and autonomy of individual practitioners

In contrast to the beliefs underlying the concept of self-governance, there is a fear that the status and autonomy of individual practitioners may be diminished by a team approach, particularly where the functions previ-ously identified with one health profession are taken over by another. This could lead to demarcation disputes. There is concern by midwives, for example, when practice nurses are permitted to undertake routine antenatal tests for women.[10] Such tensions result from a lack of confidence in one's own professional standing, from a lack of discussion about task appropriateness, and from a failure to provide the levels of training neces-sary to ensure acceptable competence. Teams do not simply grow, they need operational policies and team leadership. If these requirements are not provided, the result could be confusion, wasted resources and potential harm to patients.[9]

Purchasing issues

Whilst the 1997 White Paper abolishes the internal market, it still envisages the existence of service level agreements between various organisations providing healthcare. It will still be possible for purchasers to define, within the terms of these agreements, integrated nursing team arrangements and sanctions when these terms have not been implemented. The agreements could also denote the funds that should be allocated against team activities by the providers. NHS agreements between health service bodies are not enforceable in law, and any dispute can lead to an arbiter being set up by the Secretary of State.[11] Agreements with individuals practising as self-employed practitioners or with organisations outside the NHS are not covered by this prohibition and can be enforced through the courts.

Patients' rights: confidentiality and access to healthcare

Whilst the patient/client is concerned with the individual practitioner he or she should be made aware that confidential information may be passed between team members in the interests of the patient. If the patient requests that information be kept confidential by a particular professional e.g. that he/she has suicidal thoughts, it should be made clear to him/her that other members of the team caring for them may need to know that information in their best interests.

The patient has a statutory right of access to both personal health information and to information kept by the social services. These statutory rights derive from different legislative enactments and it is essential that when teams are formed the implications of statutory rights to access of records be considered.[12] When a unified system of record keeping is adopted the legislation under which the patient has access to these records should be clarified.

Disputes between practitioners and the involvement of the patient

Where there has been a failure in communication between team members or where there is friction over responsibilities and roles, there is a danger that the patient could be brought unwittingly into the conflict. For example, a practice nurse could visit a patient giving specific advice about a dressing. If the patient is visited by a district nurse who gives conflicting advice, and the patient says 'But the practice nurse said', the district nurse must be careful not to unnecessarily criticise the practice nurse. If the practice nurse has given negligent advice, the district nurse should arrange for the practice nurse to revisit the patient and correct the failure.[13] These are difficult interdisciplinary issues and require both professional sensitivity and the protection of patients from unsafe practice.

The future

Ensuring effective teamwork across a variety of organisations is extremely difficult, particularly when individual team members are separately employed. It is possible that the future involves new organisations for primary healthcare which become the sole employers of the entire team, with the exception of voluntary workers. The Green Paper on mental health services puts forward for discussion four specific options for purchasers of mental health services which would adjust, if necessary through legislation, the current boundaries between health and social care for people with severe mental illness.[14] If these changes do come about, they could pave the way to one of the most important developments within healthcare this century. Perhaps the 21st century will see England, Wales and Scotland following the Northern Ireland model of integrated health and social care.

References

1 Department of Health (1997) *The New NHS: modern, dependable*. The Stationery Office, London.
2 Welsh Office (1998) *Putting Patients First*. The Stationery Office, London.
3 Wilsher *v* Essex (1986). **3** *All ER* 801 (CA).
4 JM Consulting Ltd (1997) *The Regulation of Nurses, Midwives and Health Visitors*. JM Consulting Ltd, Bristol.
5 *The Medicinal Products (Nurse Prescribing etc) Act 1992*.
6 *Nurses' Formulary*: appendix to the *British National Formulary* revised each year.
7 Dimond BC (1995) *Nurse Prescribing*. Merck Dermatology and Scutari Press, London.

8 Pugsley D, Rees P and Dimond BC (1996) Community mental health teams: development in community care. *British J Nursing.* **5**(22): 1398–401.

9 Porter-O'Grady T and Kruger-Wilson C (1996) *The Leadership Revolution in Healthcare: altering systems, changing behaviour.* Aspen, Rockville, MD.

10 Dimond B (1996) When is a nurse a midwife? *Modern Midwife.* **6**(1):34–5.

11 Section 4 of the *NHS and Community Care Act 1990* prevents recourse to the courts.

12 *Access to Health Records Act 1990; Access to Personal Files Act 1987.*

13 Dimond BC (1997) *The Legal Aspects of Care in the Community.* Macmillan Press, Basingstoke.

14 Department of Health (1997) *Green Paper Developing Partnerships in Mental Health.* HMSO, London.

Further reading list

Brazier M (ed) (1988) *Street on Torts* (8th ed). Butterworths, London.

Brazier M (1992) *Medicine: patients and the law.* Penguin, London.

Clarkson CMV and Keating HM (1994) *Criminal Law: text and materials* (3rd ed). Sweet & Maxwell, London.

Dimond BC (1995) *Legal Aspects of Nursing* (2nd ed). Prentice Hall, London.

Dimond BC (1996) *Legal Aspects of Child Healthcare.* Mosby, London.

Dimond BC (1993) *Patients Rights, Responsibilities and the Nurse.* Quay Publishing, Salisbury.

Dimond BD (1994) *Legal Aspects of Midwifery.* Midwives Press, Hale, Cheshire.

Dimond BD and Barker F (1996) *Mental Health Law for Nurses.* Blackwell Science, Oxford.

Ellis N (1998) *General Practice Employment Handbook.* Radcliffe Medical Press, Oxford.

Finch J (ed) (1994) *Speller's Law Relating to Hospitals* (7th ed). Chapman and Hall Medical, London.

Kidner R (1993) *Blackstone's Statutes on Employment Law* (3rd ed). Blackstones, London.

Kloss D (1994) *Occupational Health Law* (2nd ed). Blackwell Scientific Publications, Oxford.

Knight B (1992) *Legal Aspects of Medical Practice* (5th ed). Churchill Livingstone, Edinburgh.

Miers D and Page A (1990) *Legislation* (2nd ed). Sweet & Maxwell, London.

Selwyn N (ed) (1993) *Selwyn's Law of Employment* (8th ed). Butterworths, London.

Smith K and Keenan D (eds) (1992) *Smith and Keenan English Law* (10th ed). Pitman, London.

White R, Carr P and Lowe N (1991) *A Guide to the Children Act 1989.* Butterworths, London.

Acknowledgements

I wish to acknowledge Kath Hier for her assistance in the preparation of this chapter and Denise Houghton, Executive Director of Nursing, Rochdale Healthcare NHS Trust for her guidance on the concept of 'self-governance'.

10

Future directions for primary care

Brenda Poulton

In her inaugural Henderson Memorial Lecture at the International Council of Nurses in 1997, Clark expressed her dream that nursing in the 21st century would be dominated by community nursing and primary healthcare.[1] She predicted a scenario where the information superhighway would change the delivery of healthcare 'from a system driven by the provider to one driven by the consumer'. In this brave new world community nurses would have a leading role to play in assisting patients and clients to access information, interpret it and make informed choices about their health. Envisioning the future in this way presents major challenges to all those working in primary care but in terms of nursing, Clark suggests four preconditions which will influence the ability of nursing to adapt to the future:

1 the way in which nursing is organised within the healthcare sector

2 how practice is regulated and quality is assured

3 preparation for practice

4 how nurses perceive their roles.

It would be perverse to suggest that community nursing has control over its future determination. To a large extent the organisational structure of healthcare is determined by current political philosophies and policy framework which inform the way care is delivered. Increasingly, however, the nursing voice is being heeded by policy makers. Nurses make up 85% of the NHS workforce and if they speak in unison they can, in the words of Dr Mahler, former Director General of WHO, become a 'powerhouse for change'. This chapter aims to examine differing models of primary care nursing delivery and how roles might develop in the future. Changes in professional power and increasing consumerism will be discussed in terms of their implications for integrated nursing teams (INTs) and primary care.

Putting the future into context

The late 1990s have witnessed another upheaval in healthcare organisation within the NHS. During the early part of this decade the Conservative administration introduced the internal market in an effort to make the health service 'needs driven' rather than 'professionally driven'. This had the effect of making healthcare commissioners scrutinise services more closely and look for evidence of effectiveness. The downside of the internal market was increased bureaucracy and inequity of service provision. The new Labour administration promises to rectify these problems by dismantling the internal market and subsuming general practitioner fundholding into primary care groups.[2] Such groups will build on models of good practice in primary care and reflect the requirements of local communities. It also assures that community nurses will play an equal role in shaping primary care-based services.

Alongside these proposals is the Government's commitment to improving the nation's health by addressing health needs within the wider public health context, taking into account socio-economic factors, housing, employment, air quality and safe water supplies.[3] These aims demand both an interprofessional and an interagency approach through Health Improvement Programmes and targeting of specific Health Action Zones which, although specific to England, are likely to be generic themes within the NHS.

The way nursing responds to these challenges will be influenced to some extent by nurse education. Chapter 5 examined the UKCC model of preparation of nurses for specialist practice in the community. This is based on core learning outcomes with eight specialist practitioner routes. Such courses are now provided as community nursing degree programmes throughout the UK. However, in the light of the review of the UKCC and the National Boards, the specialist practice titles may well change. For example, the review of the *Nurses, Midwives and Health Visitors' Act* proposes condensing the 15 parts of the register to six.[4] This would involve a phasing out of the registration of health visitors and voluntary recording of all community specialist practice qualifications. These changes, if they come about, would involve a total rethink of roles and titles in community nursing.

Evaluation of different models of nursing care delivery in primary care

It has been argued that developing INTs within primary care organisations would be one step closer to the bringing together of functional teams to make up a coherent whole. Although there are several examples of this concept there is very little in the way of objective evaluation of such initiatives.

The Northern and Yorkshire region evaluated a project to encourage 10 primary care teams to work in an integrated way.[5] Resources were devolved down to practice level and facilitated teams developed practice-based health needs analysis (HNA). Although all the teams worked hard to develop HNA they had difficulty translating these into objectives for practice. The aim was to involve the whole primary care team, including general practitioners. In the event the nursing teams were the driving force behind the initiative and where doctors were involved, they only played a marginal role. The biggest barrier, however, was the organisational structure of primary healthcare. Differing reward systems and multiple lines of management accountability militated against a team approach to care.

The National Health Service Executive funded a project to develop a small number of primary care teams across England, using multidisciplinary audit to encourage a team approach to care.[6] The project involved the facilitation and process evaluation of six primary care teams, using practice health profiles to set priorities for intervention. In spite of the multi-professional approach, nurses again took the lead in the project. Each practice had a practice development co-ordinator, which in each case was from a nursing background, either district, practice nursing or health visiting. The positive findings were first, that HNA is a positive way of identifying topics for change and second, the practice co-ordinator is a critical success factor for the implementation of audit. On the negative side, there was poor commitment to multidisciplinary audit in primary care. It was difficult to achieve a wide involvement in audit and ineffective collaboration between team members led to high stress levels.

The Cardiff practice-based teams project involved 12 practices where INTs were positively encouraged by making the 'attached' nurses practice-exclusive and basing them as far as possible within the same building.[7] Nursing budgets were devolved to these nursing teams who were encouraged to select their own team leader from within the nursing group. The project was evaluated in terms of benefits to patients, to the teams themselves and to general practitioners. In some cases, the integration of the nursing teams was achieved but only six of the teams opted to take on their own budget. Management functions were devolved and resulted in a higher level of satisfaction with the service. Proxy outcomes were identified which have the potential for improving patient outcomes in the future. For example, one practice developed practice-based service contracts involving the management of post-natal depression (health visitors) and wound care (district nurses). Interventions will be measured by these proxy outcomes rather than on client contacts. Another nursing team is developing an integrated approach to the prevention and management of diabetes within a Bengali population. A targeted, collaborative approach has the potential to improve the quality and cost-effectiveness of the service. Barriers that still need to be overcome are: improvement of support for needs assessment and priority setting; development of more specific patient outcomes; support to assist staff to cope with changing roles and responsibility; and the perennial problem of how to improve communication between professionals.

A more recent project, spearheaded by Hillingdon Health Authority, sought to develop extended primary care teams. These consisted of general practitioners, nurses and administrative staff and also the wider nursing service (school nurses, community mental health nurses, Macmillan nurses and midwives) as well as the paramedical specialties such as podiatry, physiotherapy and pharmacy. The evaluation demonstrated improved communication within the extended team and much closer working between practice and attached nursing staff.[8]

In terms of INTs, the messages for the future are:

- to facilitate more co-ordinated services, the differing lines of management and accountability need to be addressed
- INTs need to have budgetary and management control
- a health needs analysis of the defined population forms a basis for setting practice
- the process needs careful facilitation
- evaluation of the process, audit and feedback need to be included
- service users need to be involved at every stage in the process.

Changing organisation of primary healthcare

The World Health Organisation (WHO) philosophy of primary healthcare emphasises the principles of community participation, equity of provision

based on intersectoral collaboration between communities and other services, e.g. health, social services and housing.[9] This model goes far beyond
the individualistic approach of primary medical care as outlined by Ashton
and Seymour: 'a medical concept based on the equitable availability and
accessibility of good quality preventive and treatment services from a team
of health workers based in the community'.[10]

At its inception the National Health Service aimed to eliminate
Beveridge's five giants – squalor, disease, idleness, want and ignorance.[11]
The Government has reaffirmed its commitment to such an approach in
the Green Paper on public health in which it pledges to 'tackle the root
causes of ill health by establishing a contract for health', addressing issues
at policy, organisational and individual behavioural levels.[3]

In the future it is envisaged that primary care teams will deliver more
community orientated care. Although some commentators may disagree,
there is evidence to show a clear relationship between public health and
general medical practice. Over two decades ago, Tudor Hart coined the
term 'inverse care law' to describe the trend for poorer provision of care in
areas of high need.[12] This population-based approach has become known
as 'community orientated primary healthcare' and involves integrating
personal care with an epidemiological assessment of needs.[13-16] This fits
in well with initiatives such as the Health Action Zones, which involve
partnerships between local health providers, local authorities, community
groups, the voluntary sector and local businesses.

In a major study of teamworking in primary care it was concluded that
in order to achieve more collaboration, the different lines of management
responsibility and accountability need to be dismantled and that team
members should be subject to the same reward systems.[17] The *Primary Care
Act* put in place the necessary legislation to allow such developments and
paved the way towards salaried medical and nursing practitioners working as equal partners in practice.[18]

A range of pilot schemes has been set up and around 100 schemes in
England and Scotland will start in April 1998. Of these, six are nurse-led
and two involve nurse–general practitioner partnerships. The nurse-led
pilots tend to focus on patient groups such as the homeless and 'travellers'
whose needs have been neglected by traditional services.[19] Although the
Primary Care Act enables more innovative skill-mixes in primary care,
there are still constraints that militate against nurses taking a more leading
role in primary care. Despite the difficulties recruiting general practitioners
to inner city areas, the bureaucratic process (and professional hurdles)
involved in setting up nurse-led pilots have caused many problems.[20]

Perhaps we can predict that not only will there be less general practitioners in the future, but that many will be women wishing to combine a

career with a family life and for whom a salaried service will be more attractive. It could well be that although the independent contractual status of general practitioners is held dear, this contract will become less attractive and may automatically evaporate if primary care trusts emerge.

Changing roles

The crux of making INTs work is to accept that teamworking is about sharing skills and not about preserving nursing roles which have suited professional groupings. There is confusion as to what constitutes specialist nursing practice. As Kelly suggests, 'assertions of specialist knowledge and skills gained through education do not provide empirical proof of professional expertise', and there is pressure on the UKCC to recognise nurse practitioners within the post-registration community nursing specialist programme.[21] But these professional arguments do nothing to help the establishment of integrated nursing. Gardener warns against territoriality and says 'health visiting doesn't matter ... district nursing doesn't matter ... practice nursing doesn't matter ... nurse practitioners don't matter ... what matters is people'.[22] In the future, the skills to meet the needs of primary care will be more important than titles.[23]

Power and professionalism

It is impossible to ignore the unequal power base between doctors and other members of the primary care team. In early studies of teamwork in primary care McIntosh and Dingwell suggested that for nurses, 'if partnership with doctors exists at all, it can be best described as *junior partnership'.*[24] Although made 20 years ago, the comments remain pertinent. General practitioners are, in effect, small businessmen who remain in control of their practice and 'own' the list population. Many practice nurses find that the employer/employee situation makes it difficult for them to contribute on an equal basis, and attached nurses felt that fundholding contracts gave general practitioners control over their work. There is also a powerful gender issue in that the unequal power structures between doctors and nurses reflect the unequal power relationships between men and women in contemporary society. Despite women forming the largest proportion of the healthcare workforce, according to Osborne, male patterns of accountability continue to dominate the service.[25]

Salvage suggests that the female predominance in nursing, compounded by the fact that nurses, particularly in primary care, work part-time, gives the workforce a very weak negotiation position regarding wages.[26]

The Primary Care Act Pilots open the way for nurse/general practitioner partnerships, provided nurses are willing to take on the risk and accountability responsibilities involved. Some general practitioners may argue that nurses lack the knowledge and skills to cope with the myriad of problems encountered in general practice. But the trends clearly indicate that the primary care skill-mix for the future will involve all practitioners – be they general practitioners, nurses, professions allied to medicine, social workers and the wider group of people who contribute to the health of the community.

Increasing consumerism

Successive government policy directives have endorsed the involvement of consumers in shaping healthcare. Consumer involvement involves a broad range of relationships and ranges from simple information giving, through consultation and establishing consumer satisfaction, to, at the ultimate level, sharing the decision-making processes, often referred to as empowerment.[27] The most frequent method of consumer involvement in primary care is the evaluation of patient satisfaction with services.[28] Such surveys tend to examine the professional rather than the consumer agenda although there is a wealth of evidence to show that these two agendas may differ.[29,30] The satisfaction literature is mostly based on studies of the doctor–patient interactions, very few have addressed interactions with other professionals in primary care.[27] Yet, if we are to move to a team approach to care it is essential that the consumer view of this is carefully assessed.

When a questionnaire designed to evaluate general practitioner consultations was adapted for use with nursing contacts it was found that patients rated nurses as being more thorough in their assessment and more willing to listen to the patient's own perceptions of their illness.[31,32] Patients rated general practitioners higher on 'depth of relationship'. It has also been demonstrated that patients generally accept the nurse practitioner role and are happy to see a nurse rather than a doctor for some conditions.[33] More work, including qualitative ways of evaluating patient perceptions, is required to validate these findings.[8]

The involvement of local communities in assessing their health needs is less well developed. Rapid participatory appraisal is a technique used in developing countries and incorporates semi-structured interviews and focus groups of key informants in the community to assess priorities, often in relation to deprived communities and as a method of involving users in producing general practice population profiles.[34-37]

Patient participation groups are often criticised because they often attract an unrepresentative articulate middle class, who restrict their activities to fundraising and the provision of transport and prescription services for the housebound. It is not an easy task to obtain appropriate lay involvement. Joule, when considering involvement in audit, identified three main constraints.[38] First, healthcare is seen as too technical for lay people to understand. Second, issues of confidentiality are raised and, third, groups of people are only deemed competent to comment on areas perceived to be within their remit, e.g. people from ethnic groups are only allowed to comment on cultural issues.

Clearly, achieving involvement demands an acceptance that those consumers understand, and have a valid opinion about, healthcare services. Perhaps courses for consumer members of primary care commissioning groups will be required, in the same way that training is provided for parent school governors. The National Association of Patient Participation Groups (NAPP) is actively promoting a new generation of consumers willing to become more involved in health planning. They will be more knowledgeable and active in shaping the health service than their predecessors. This consumer empowerment will inevitably challenge the professional protectionism of primary care practitioners.

Integrated nursing teams in the future

The current political imperative emphasises the importance of a public health approach that requires both an interprofessional and intersectoral approach. The climate is therefore ripe for the provision of a range of services in the community. Could an urban Primary Care Centre be open around the clock? Could it provide a range of services, general medical services, direct access generalist nurse practitioners, as well as more specialised services such as chronic disease management, womens' health and complementary therapies? For people in more rural areas, telephone advice systems, supported by nurses and general practitioners will be available. Anything seems likely now that the knots, which bound up the professional structures in primary care, have been loosened.

The interface between medicine and nursing will be less well defined, but delegation and substitution, driven by doctors or managers and perceived as a cost-saving exercise, will cause problems. There is no doubt that there will be a blurring of nursing roles, not so much a generic community nurse but the perpetuation of skill-sharing and role development to meet community needs.

All of which implies that integrated nursing teams represent merely a stage in the development of more integrated primary care. Teamwork has been a maligned term and the primary care organisation of the future will be much too large to make up a realistic 'team' in the true sense of the term. Primary care organisations will need to be grouped into functional groups defined to a much greater extent by consumers. There is clearly a long way to go yet.

References

1   Clark Dame J (1998) The unique function of the nurse. *Nursing Standard.* **12**(16):39–42.
2   Department of Health (1997) *The New NHS: modern, dependable.* The Stationery Office, London.
3   Department of Health (1998) *Our Healthier Nation: a contract for health* (consultation document). The Stationery Office, London.
4   JM Consulting Ltd (1997) *The Regulation of Nurses, Midwives and Health Visitors.* JM Consulting Ltd, Bristol.
5   West MA, Poulton BC and Hardy G (1994) *New Models of Primary Care: The Northern & Yorkshire Region Micropurchasing Project.* NHSE Northern & Yorkshire, Harrogate.
6   Poulton BC (1996) *Multidisciplinary Audit in Primary Healthcare.* Daphne Heald Research Unit, Royal College of Nursing, London.
7   Poulton BC (1997) *Evaluation of Cardiff Community Healthcare Practice-based Teams Project.* Daphne Heald Research Unit, Royal College of Nursing, London.
8   Poulton BC (1997) *Joint Ventures Initiative for Primary Care Team Development in Hillingdon.* Royal College of Nursing, London.
9   World Health Organisation (1978) The Alma-Ata Conference on Primary Healthcare. *WHO Chronicle.* **32**.
10 Ashton J and Seymour H (1988) *The New Public Health.* Open University Press, Buckingham.
11 Beveridge Sir W (1942) *Social Insurance and Allied Services* (Cmd 6404, 6405). HMSO, London.
12 Tudor Hart J (1971) The Inverse Care Law. *Lancet.* **I**:405–12.
13 Abrahamson JH (1988) Community orientated primary care: strategy, approaches and practice. *Public Health Review* (Israel). **16**:35–8.

14   Epstein L and Eshed H (1988) Community orientated primary health-care. *South African Med J.* **73**:220–3.

15   Frome PS (1989) Is community orientated primary care a viable concept in actual practice? *J Family Practice.* **28**:203–8.

16   Gillam S, Pampling D, McClenahan J et al. (1994) *Community Orientated Primary Care.* King's Fund, London.

17   Poulton BC (1995) *Effective Multidisciplinary Teamwork in Primary Healthcare* (dissertation). Institute of Work Psychology, University of Sheffield. Unpublished.

18   Health Departments of Great Britain (1996) *Choice and Opportunity: primary care. The future.* HMSO, London.

19   Gulland A (1998) Revving up for life in the pilot seat. *Nursing Times.* **94**(1):14–15.

20   Kenny C (1998) Nice idea, shame about the pace. *Nursing Times.* **94**(1):15.

21   Kelly A (1996) The concept of the specialist community nurse. *J Advanced Nursing.* **24**:42–52.

22   Gardner L (1998) Leading primary care: time for action. *Health Visitor.* **71**(1):21–2.

23   Poulton BC (1994) *A needs-based approach to developing and evaluating the nurse practitioner role.* Paper presented at the Second International Nurse Practitioner Conference, 5–7 August.

24   McIntosh J and Dingwall R (1978) Teamwork in theory and practice. In: R Dingwall and J McIntosh (eds) *Readings in the Sociology of Nursing.* Churchill Livingstone, Edinburgh.

25   Osborne K (1991) Women's work… is never done. In: J Firth-Couzens and MA West (eds) *Women and Work: psychological and organizational perspectives.* Open University Press, Buckingham.

26   Salvage J (1985) *The Politics of Nursing.* Heinemann, London.

27   Poulton BC (1997) Consumer feedback and determining satisfaction with services. In: C Mason (ed) *Qualitative Issues in Community Health-care Nursing.* Macmillan, Basingstoke.

28   McIver S (1993) *Obtaining the Views of Users of Primary and Community Healthcare Services.* King's Fund Centre, London.

29   Smith C and Armstrong D (1989) Comparison of criteria derived by government and patients for evaluating general practitioner services. *BMJ.* **299**:494–6.

30   Al-Bashir M and Armstrong D (1991) Preferences of healthy and ill patients for the style of general practitioner care: implications for workload and financial incentives. *British J Gen Prac.* **41**:6–8.

31   Baker R (1990) Development of a questionnaire to assess patients' satisfaction with consultation in general practice. *British J Gen Prac.* **40**: 487–90.

32 Poulton BC (1996) Use of the consultation satisfaction questionnaire to examine patients' satisfaction with general practitioners and community nurses: reliability, replicability and discriminant validity. *British J Gen Prac.* **46**:26–31.

33 Poulton BC (1995) Keeping the customer satisfied. *Primary Health Care.* **5**(4):16–19.

34 Vuori H (1986) Community participation in primary healthcare: a means to an end. In: H Vuori and JEF Hastings (eds) *Patterns of Community Participation in Primary Healthcare.* WHO, Copenhagen.

35 Doyle N (1993) Workshop 4: models of lay participation. In: M Dunning and G Needham (eds) *But Will It Work Doctor? Report of a conference about involving users in health services outcomes research.* King's Fund Centre, London.

36 Ong BN, Humphris G, Annett H *et al.* (1991) Rapid appraisal in an urban setting: an example from the developed world. *Soc Sci Med.* **32**(8):909–15.

37 Murray SA, Tapson J, Turnbull L *et al.* (1994) Listening to local voices: adapting rapid appraisal to assess health and social need in general practice. *BMJ.* **308**:698–700.

38 Joule N (1992) *User Involvement in Medical Audit.* Greater London Association of Community Health Councils, London.

Index

access to healthcare 108
accountability
  future changes 21
  legal issues 103
  male patterns 118
  Oxfordshire approach 93, 98
accreditation 22
administration role of nurses 72
advantages of integrated nursing
      teams 44
agency, substitution of 19, 21, 22, 23
ageing of population 14
assessment, nursing 72
attached staff 38, 42, 82, 115
audit
  clinical 22
  nursing 72
autonomy 21, 107

Bevan, Aneurin 79
Birchwood Medical Centre,
      Warrington 42
Boer War 8
budgets *see* financial issues
BUPA primary care centres 10

'care partners', changes 17
carers for dependent relatives 17
case law 101
case management 73
centres for complementary therapies
      10
Charters 14, 16, 17
clinical audit 22
clinical governance 22, 32
Code of Professional Conduct 30

collaboration, interagency 19, 23
collectivist approach to healthcare 15
commissioning
  legal issues 108
  locality 10, 45–6, 81, 83
  marginalisation and involvement
      33, 34
  White Paper proposals 32, 45
common law 101
communication 40, 106
community care 20–2
community care centres 9, 10
community development agencies 9
community healthcare nurses
      (CHCNs)
  Cumberlege Report 39
  development 42–3, 80–1
  employment status 38
  future 55–7, 113–14
  marginalisation and involvement
      issues 33
  new NHS 31
  new public health 34
  Oxfordshire approach 91–3, 98
    decision making 97
    devolved budgets 94–6, 97–8
    funding 94
  power inequalities 79
  primary healthcare teams,
      limitations 81
  roles 67, 70
  teamwork 57–8, 83
community hospitals 20
community psychiatric nurses 45
complementary therapy centres 10
conditions of employment 106

confidentiality 108, 120
consortia 9, 10
consumerism 14, 119–20
contracts, nurses' 21–2
co-ordinated professional teams
    (CPTs) 46
co-ordinators, practice development
    115
core team model 43
corporatism 22
cost-benefit data 16
cost-effectiveness data 16
counselling skills 72
Crimean War 8
Cumberlege Report 39, 82

day surgery 21
decision making, Oxfordshire
    approach 97
delegation
    legal issues 105, 107
    and skill-mix 61, 62
    see also substitution, healthcare
demarcation disputes 107
development of integrated nursing
    teams 42–4
devolved budgets 94–6
    cost effectiveness 97–8
disadvantages of integrated nursing
    teams 44–5
district general hospitals (DGHs)
    patterns of healthcare provision
        17–18
    substitution, healthcare 19, 20
district nurses
    Oxfordshire approach 92
    prescribing 104
    training issues 56
    see also community healthcare nurses
diversification 61–2

education see training issues
effectiveness in healthcare
    information on 16
    prioritisation 15
    teamwork 46–7

efficiency in healthcare
    government policy 15
    information on 16
electronic data interchange 15–16
emergence of integrated nursing
    teams 37–9
employment conditions 106
empowerment 119–20
European Convention on Human
    Rights 101
evidence-based practice 16
examples of integrated nursing teams
    83–7
extended primary care teams 116

facilitation of nursing teams 58–9,
    60, 68
financial issues 4, 91–4, 98–9
    accountability 98
    community nursing budgets 45
        devolved 94–6, 97–8
    decision making 97
    fundholding 39–40
    funding integrated nursing teams
        94
    government expenditure 14–15
    legal aspects 107, 108
    substitution, healthcare 21, 22, 23
Four Elms Medical Centre, Cardiff 42,
    86
fundholding 1
    dismantling 32
    and working relationship 39–40
future directions for primary care 4–5,
    109, 113–14, 120–1
    consumerism 119–20
    contextualising the future 114
    evaluation of nursing models
        115–16
    organisation of primary care 116–18
    power and professionalism 118–19
    roles, changes in 118
    and substitution, healthcare 21

gender issues 118
generalism vs. specialism 1

General Medical Services (GMS) 94
general practitioner commissioning
    group pilots 10
governance, clinical 22, 32
governments
    'care partners', changes 17
    NHS changes 15, 16, 31–2, 114
    primary care-led NHS 29
    societal changes 14–15
    see also political and policy context
GP commissioning group pilots 10
growth of integrated nursing teams 3,
    79–81, 87–8

Health Action Zones 10, 114, 117
Health CALL primary care centres 10
health centres 81
Health Improvement Plan 32
Health Improvement Programmes 114
health needs analysis (HNA) 68–9,
    115, 119–20
health parks 10
health visitors
    emergence 80
    future 114
    legal issues 104
    Oxfordshire approach 92
    training issues 56, 80
    see also community healthcare
        nurses
Healthy Living Centres 10
Heathrow Debate 31
Hillfields, Coventry 87
Hospital and Community Health
    Services (HCHS) 94
hospital trust primary care units 10
Human Rights Bill 1997 101

information
    on effectiveness 16
    on efficiency 16
    in new NHS 32
    about patients 16
    for patients 16
information technology (IT) 15–16, 19
infrastructure, nurses' lack of 33

insurance for legal proceedings 103
interagency collaboration 19, 23
interprofessional education 63
interprofessional rivalry 16
introductory group working 60, 61
inverse care law 117
involvement issues 33–4

joint funding 17
judge-made law 101
junior doctors 19

key workers 103

labour market context of integrated
    nursing teams 30–1
Ladies' Sanitary Reform Association
    80
leadership, team 44, 74–7
    legal issues 102
    Oxfordshire approach 92
legal issues 4, 101
    communication 106
    delegation and supervision 105
    disputes between practitioners
        108–9
    employment conditions 106
    future 109
    individual accountability 103
    key workers 103
    managerial control and hierarchy
        105–6
    nurse prescribing 104
    patients' rights 108
    purchasing issues 108
    scope of professional practice 104
    self-managing team concept 106–7
    status and autonomy of individual
        practitioners 107
    statutory framework and primary
        healthcare 101–2
    team liability 102
    training and professional
        development 105
liability 102, 103, 104
listening skills 72

Llyn y fran Practice, Cardiganshire 85–6
locality commissioning groups 10, 45–6, 81, 83
locational substitution 18, 19, 21, 22, 23
Lyme Regis Community Care Unit 42

management 4, 91–4, 98–9
  accountability 98
  decision making 97
  legal issues 105–6
  maternity leave cover 97
  sickness cover 97
  skills 92
  substitution, healthcare 22
managers, nurse 74, 91, 93
marginalisation issues 33–4
maternity leave cover, Oxfordshire approach 97
medical records
  access to 108
  shared 73
mental health services 109
midwives 4
multidisciplinary education 62–3
multinational companies, teamwork questioned by 41
multiskilling 30

National Association of Patient Participation Groups (NAPP) 120
National Health Service, changes 15–16, 31–2
National Health Service Act 1946 79, 80
National Health Service and Community Care Act 1990 101–2
National Health Service (Primary Care) Act 1997 7, 102, 117
National Insurance Act 1911 7–8, 79
neighbourhood nursing teams (NNTs) 82

New NHS, The (1997 White Paper) 22, 45
nurse managers 74, 91, 93
nurse practitioners
  ascendancy 29
  development of role 45
  patients' acceptance 119
  progress of concept 82
nurse prescribing 55, 72, 82, 104
Nurses Act 1925 80
Nurses' Formulary 104
Nurses, Midwives and Health Visitors' Act, review 114

one-stop shop concept 46
organisation of primary care, changes 1–2, 7–11, 114, 116–18

pastoral care centres 10
patients
  consumerism 119–20
  involvement in disputes 108–9
  participation groups 120
  rights 108
pilot practices 7, 8, 10
planning
  by consumers 120
  by nurses 22
  of teams 48
political and policy context 2, 27–8, 35
  integrated nursing teams and primary care, redefinition 28–9
  marginalisation and involvement issues 33–4
  new NHS 31–2
  new public health 34
  professional and labour market context 30–1
post-operative care 21
post-registration education and practice (PREP) 56, 57, 104, 105, 118
poverty, impact on health 34
power and professionalism 118–19
practice development co-ordinators 115

practice nurses
  ascendancy 29
  employment status 38, 82
  marginalisation and involvement
    issues 33
  Oxfordshire approach 92, 94
  primary healthcare non-teams 39
  staff substitutions 19, 21
  training issues 56
Premier Community Trust,
  Stoke-on-Trent 42
Premier Health Trust, South
  Staffordshire 86
prescribing, nurse 55, 72, 82
  legal issues 104
primary care, impact of substitution
  on 20–2
Primary Care Act 1996 29
primary care agencies 9
primary care centres 10
Primary Care: delivering the future (1996
  White Paper) 62
primary care groups (PCGs) 99
  commissioning 32
  marginalisation and involvement
    33, 34
  pilots 10
  planning and management of teams
    48
primary healthcare, definitions 28–9
primary healthcare non-teams 39–40
primary healthcare teams (PHCTs) 81
  decision making 91
  and integrated nursing teams:
    integral vs. alternative 2–3, 50
  advantages and disadvantages of
    integrated nursing teams 44–5
  attempted solutions 41–2
  barriers to teamwork 40–1
  building effective teams in the
    future 46–7
  emergence of integrated nursing
    teams 37–9
  managed primary care
    organisation, development
    42–4

new NHS 45–6
  planned and managed teams,
    implications for integrated
    nursing teams 48–9
  primary healthcare non-teams
    39–40
  weaknesses 27
primary medical services pilots 10
private sector 17, 21
professional context of integrated
  nursing teams 30–1
professional development see training
  issues
professionalism and power 118–19
professional self-regulation 32
Project 2000 56
public demands and expectations 14
public health, new 34
purchasing see commissioning

quality in healthcare
  assurance 46
  monitoring 22, 46
  prioritisation 15

records
  access to 108
  shared 73
'Red Book' 1
re-engineering 30, 46
referrals 73
reprofiling 30
resource centres 10
risk management 22
rivalry, inter-professional 16
roles of nurses in integrated teams 3,
    67–72, 73–4, 77
  administration or prescribing 72
  assessment, nursing 72
  audit, nursing 72
  changes 118
  counselling skills 72
  expansion 30, 104
  planning 22
  referral and case management 73
  shared records and guidelines 73

supervision and professional
    development 73
    team leadership 74–7
Roy Report 67

salaried GP service 1, 46
school nurses 56
Scope of Professional Practice 30, 104
'seamless' care 19
seconded teams 84, 87
self-governance 107
self-managed teams 84, 86
    legal issues 106–7
    Oxfordshire approach 91, 92–4, 98–9
self-regulation, professional 32
shared records and guidelines 73
shared skills 69–70
sickness cover, Oxfordshire approach
    97
skill-mix 70–1
    reviews 30
    training issues 60–2
skill-sharing 30
'smart cards' 15–16
social context of health 34
social exclusion, impact on health 34
social services
    changes 17
    substitution, healthcare 19, 21, 23
society, changes 14–15
specialism
    development of roles 45
    future 114, 118
    vs. generalism 1
specific practice focus teams 84
specific skills 70
staff substitutions 19, 21, 22, 23
Statement of Fees and Allowances 1
status of practitioners 107
statutory framework 101–2
statutory law 101
stomach ulcers 19
stress levels 98
substitution, healthcare 2, 13,
    17–20, 24
    appropriateness 22–3

changing world 13–14
    'care partners' 17
    NHS 15–16
    society 14–15
    impact on primary care and
        community nursing 20–2
    and skill-mix 61
supervision of nurses 73
supervision 105

team leadership 44, 74–7
    legal issues 102
    Oxfordshire 92
teamwork
    barriers 40–1, 43
    community nursing 57–8
    difficulties 39
    effective 46–7
    facilitation 58–9, 60, 68
    fact vs. fiction 82–3
    and fundholding 40
    nurses' commitment to 44, 57
    see also primary healthcare teams
technology
    changes within NHS 15, 32
    information technology 15–16, 19
    substitutions 19, 21, 22, 23
telemedicine 19
Thornton Medical Centre, Lancashire
    84–5
Tile Hill, Coventry 86–7
total purchasing pilots 10
training issues 3–4, 63–4
    community nurses 55–7
    facilitation 58–9
    identifying needs 59–60, 73
    legal aspects 105
    multidisciplinary 62–3
    scope 55
    skill-mix in primary care 60–2
    teamworking ethos 57–8

ulcers, stomach 19
United Kingdom Central Council for
    Nursing, Midwifery and Health
    Visiting (UKCC) 55–6, 104, 118

vacancy factor 94–5
vicarious liability 103, 104
voluntary sector
 changes 17
 legal issues 103
 substitution, healthcare 19, 21

wage negotiations 119
Wemsum Valley Medical Practice,
 Norwich 42
Winch Lane Surgery, Haverfordwest 85
World Health Organisation (WHO)
 116–17